The Gray Ribbon Warrior

Theresa Catt

ISBN 978-1-63844-270-7 (paperback)
ISBN 978-1-63844-271-4 (digital)

Christian Faith Publishing, Inc.
832 Park Avenue
Meadville, PA 16335
www.christianfaithpublishing.com

Printed in the United States of America

In memory of Jesse Shane Brown
June 11, 1997–August 30, 2018

A heart full of adventure and love, a son, a brother, a friend,
a young warrior, and an inspiration to many

Everyone's story is different. I've never been the one to get the party started. This is my journey and just one part of my story. I pray yours is full of love, hope, and faith.

It's autumn, and I love this time of year. It's all about change.

Change is not only an important step in life, but it can be a very "positive affliction" cast on us whether we think we want it or not. Autumn serves to remind us that beauty and adventure can happen in change; then it follows with a time of rest. Meditation of the soul, remembering the things we have done, and then moving forward into what is yet to come...

I am the first to admit that the unknown can be a scary thing, and yes, there are moments I let it get to me. But without change, we would not see the colors of our lives, smell the excitement our souls so deeply crave, or anticipate the adventures that follow the rest.

It is important to remember—and embrace—the necessity of rest. A "winter" of reflection and time to heal so we can progress. Not all reflection needs to be caught below snowdrifts and icy winds of regret. We can rise to the challenge and let our memories glimmer brightly, like the morning sunrise reflecting off the dew on the brilliantly colored autumn leaves.

Today, however, it is not winter; so I will gather my autumn strength in all its color and glory...and I will strive to be the change that is needed.

I had been in Reno, Nevada, with my husband for a convention when we got the call that his nineteen-year-old son, Jesse, had cancer. Sarcoma. Again. This time, it was in his lung. He had lost his leg from the knee down due to the treatments and infection that followed cancer treatment when he was about nine years old.

The next few days were very unstable and stressful, so I ended up taking the car I had borrowed and driving on home to New Mexico to see if there was anything I could do. After having been away from home for several weeks, I hoped to be able to help Jesse if I could. I also just wanted at least one day in my own bed. About thirty-six hours was pretty much all I had before I headed on the twenty-four-hour or so drive back to Washington. I had to return the borrowed vehicle and pick up my daughter for our flight back to New Mexico from Washington. I was unaware then of what was actually going on in my body and why every day had felt like such a struggle.

My daughter battles with severe anxiety and is diagnosed with Asperger's Syndrome. What she is, is a smart and beautiful human being and a very talented artist. She had been living with my mother across town from us for the last few years for her to learn to live more independently. She and I had been nearly inseparable since her birth. But Tony and I moved from Washington, and she and I were both excited for her to get down to her new home with me and her stepdad. She also had plans to go back to school. College! We even talked about starting a business with her art so that she could bring in a bit of money to help cover her bills and go on the adventures she wanted.

This all sounds so simple, but it's not for a person with her diagnosis. Anxiety can be worse than any other disease because for many, it's a forever challenge. A lot of love and prayer goes into this life. So many people had asked over the years why I wasn't mad at God. I never even related to that.

After about thirty-six hours back home, I called the hospital once again, and the nurse told me that Jesse's mother and sister were still there with him and didn't want me there. A tough call. I didn't want to intrude on their family time, but I didn't know what was going on with Jesse. After a lot of prayer and crying, I got up early one morning and left the little oil-field town where we had been living for several months. I tried to get a good bit of road behind me before it got too hot. I had a long drive ahead of me to get to my daughter.

I made it to Albuquerque about five hours from home. After a short break, I was back on the road. From there, I had only made it about forty miles when the car started having trouble. I pulled over on the side of the road, afraid to cause any damage to the car, and contacted the car's owner. We decided I would have the car towed back to Albuquerque, the only realistic place nearby to find a mechanic who could work on the Audi. I called the towing company that the insurance company recommended. Dispatch said that they were going to be there in about forty-five minutes. I don't recall the exact temperature; but I believe during my wait, it hit about 112.

A police officer stopped about an hour and a half after I had been sitting there and asked if I needed a tow. I let him know I was waiting for one already. He had a small bottle of warm water and offered it to me. I was already so hot that I was grateful to have it. He left me the phone number to the police station and told me to go back about a mile and pull up to the substation parking lot. (Go figure. I'd been sitting that close to "help" for that long already! Then again, I had not realized that I was on reservation land.) Then the police officer went on his way. After a few more hours of sitting in the hot sun and starting to feel very sick, I decided to try the engine.

It started and sounded okay; so I carefully cut across the median between highways, turned around, went about a mile back, and pulled up to the gated substation parking lot. Then I found a shaded spot under a tree, let the tow company know, and continued waiting. By then, I had let my mother know that I was okay but that I was likely going to be delayed. After two more hours had passed, and a few people coming out to the car and interrogating my intentions for sitting there (but with no one offering suggestions or help), I finally pulled the car back out to the road at their urging. There was still no sign of the tow truck, and I really wasn't doing well; so I decided to try and drive it back to Albuquerque.

I drove it slowly with hazard lights on and just kept telling myself that I would be there soon and to just ignore the angry drivers. I was in the right lane, and traffic was pretty light that day; so it was the best I could do. I had a conversation with God to help calm my nerves and to not worry over heat exhaustion. He'd see me through this.

I arrived in town and finished making plans with the mechanics an hour later. I then made phone reservations and walked into a small hotel with my hair and shirt drenched with sweat. I explained my situation and got myself a room. A shower and a nap were all I wanted The clerk kindly handed me two bottles of ice-cold water, and then I headed to the room, turned on the fan, and collapsed on the worn bed.

I spent the next few days doing a lot of nothing but waiting. The Audi dealership was the only one with a mechanic able to deal with the car problems, and they had to order the part. Overall, I spent four days there. On the second day, they told me they had ordered the wrong part, and it was going to be two more days. On the fourth day, I had to check out of the hotel. I had, had enough of sitting in the room anyway, so I decided to walk to the mall down the road and see a movie with my last little bit of spare money.

It was really hot, so I wore light clothing. I enjoyed the walk; but as I turned into the mall entry, I heard a lot of activity going on around me. The sidewalk along the mall was parallel to the cars coming and going. I heard shuffling feet, talking, and a lot of laughter, which I had assumed at the time were from teenagers walking behind me. I remembered hearing the playful sounds.

The next thing I knew, I was trying to sit up on the sidewalk. Later, I had told my husband and others that I hadn't seen anything, that I just remembered the talking and laughing and felt a slight push on my shoulder. The next thing I remembered was just trying to sit up and wiping blood from all over my face. I had fallen straight forward, causing several cuts and scrapes on my face; and at the time, I felt certain that I had broken my nose. I sat there, dizzy and a bit dazed, trying to look around. I saw no one except the cars going past me.

Later that day, I recalled some of the passengers holding out their phones toward me. I assumed they were taking pictures. As for the laughing people and the pushing that I remembered feeling, I couldn't find evidence to support that as there was no one around, on foot, to be seen.

I had to sit for a few minutes to recompose myself and to try to keep myself from reacting out of embarrassment. With so much pain, I tried, unsuccessfully, to hold back the tears. After a few minutes, I pulled myself up and tried to hide the gashes and my bloody face behind my hands while I struggled to figure out what to do. The hotel had been kind enough to hold my luggage behind the counter while I went to the movie, knowing that I was still waiting on the mechanic to fix the car. I decided to go back there and get out of the heat...and out of view from the public.

As I walked in, I heard several gasps, and the clerks both stepped out to see if they could help me (and perhaps to shield me from the view of other customers). I just wanted to get cleaned up, so I asked if they had anything that I could clean my face with. They had nothing but the soap and paper towels in the restroom, so I went in and began cleaning up the mess that was my face. One of the clerks brought me ice, and I found an ibuprofen in my purse. I called a taxi to take me to the mechanic's shop and sat down in a corner near the front desk.

The taxi finally showed up about an hour and a half later to take me to the auto shop. I was going to wait there as I had already checked out from the hotel. I brought my bags and kept them nearby in the waiting room. Strangers stared while the shop employees asked if they could get me coffee or water, and in all honesty, I could see that my messed-up face made them all nervous. They hurried up the process and got the car done. One customer even asked if I had impetigo. A mechanic came out and handed me the keys; then I signed for the payment and went on my way.

As much as my face and head hurt, I was so grateful to be back in the car, no longer the spectacle. I didn't want to stop, but I still had at least twenty hours of driving ahead of me. I had decided to head to my friend's home in Nevada, visit for a day or two, and get some relaxation before heading the rest of the way up to Washington.

It was not until much later when I had already arrived home, in New Mexico, a few weeks after the fall that I still felt something was wrong. So I went to the emergency room.

This was where my journey began being documented on Facebook. It's not something I think many people would do; but my head was not clear, and my soul felt as if it was overflowing. So I wrote.

Tess
Albuquerque
July 26, 2016

I'm still trying to smile. I promise! But ya have to admit there comes a point when we question the universe…was I Genghis Kahn in my former life?

The dealership put in a defective part, so I was stuck in Albuquerque another day or two while they replaced it.

Some kids got a wee bit careless in their fun. And I met Mr. Sidewalk up close and personal. (I don't plan to repeat that blind date!) He left me plenty to remember him by… I was plucking bits of cement out of my lip and nose for the rest of the evening.

I still haven't figured out if my nose is broken or not, and I had to use a straw to drink my meal.

But it could have been worse…the US political nominations could be on *every* channel!

I so deserve a mani/pedi tomorrow!

*****

Since that posting on Facebook, it had been determined by my oncologist and Tony that it was a tumor recreating a story in my mind to explain what had happened, blending it with the noises of people I was hearing in passing cars. They said that I didn't see anyone walking or running from my incident because there was no one to see. It is amazing what the brain can do because I genuinely remembered feeling a push on my back. Maybe it was my guardian angel. Perhaps it is the power of the brain.

I headed straight to Nevada to visit my girlfriend and her family for a few days before heading on up to Washington to get my daughter.

*****

Tess
Henderson, Nevada
July 28, 2016

Some much-needed R&R time before their pool party this afternoon!

(PS. Adelle didn't want me to feel alone with my bad face; so a few stickers, and she made herself look like me. A child's perspective, genuine love and joy, is sometimes all we need to muster our strength!)

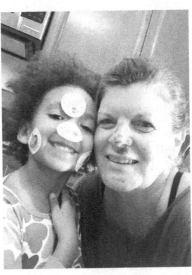

*****

I continued my daily blog writing on Facebook. Since before the fall, I had made the commitment to myself to be positive and bring that positive encouragement to others. Now more than ever,

I needed to be encouraging, to try and reach people the only way I know how. Writing was getting more difficult, but I was thinking that maybe it had to do with being tired. I was hurting; but nothing I took could shake off the dizziness, nausea, or headaches, all of which I had assumed were caused by sinus issues. I did my best to relax for a couple of days before heading on the rest of the drive to Washington State.

Tess
July 29, 2016

Friday's Tessism:

I truly believe that everything in life that happens to us, provides opportunity to make something positive.

I'm not saying it will be easy; but for example, when adversity hits, and you find that some friends back away, and maybe even are careful to not be seen connected to you until it all blows over... It's up to me (and you) to understand their fears, and forgo judgment. While that is easier said than done, it allows me (and you) to maintain dignity. Grace under fire.

Life will go on no matter how we react to it; but your strength, commitment, and compassion will allow you to shine above that adversity.

After all, it is adversity, they say, that shows who your true friends are. But adversity also allows you and me to show our humanity.

*****

Try as we may, we will never really be able to control other people's actions. We can only control our own; and sometimes, even that is hard to do. In order to do that in a positive and constructive way, we need to put certain behaviors into action every day. If we make it a habit to complain constantly, we will revert to negative reaction when adversity hits. But if we make it a habit to speak thoughtfully to others and think positively about as much as possible each day, it will most likely become our go-to reaction without even thinking about it. Adversity comes in many forms, but rarely is it ever convenient.

I was going to be positive about my experience at the sidewalk no matter what! So my solution at the time was to focus on human beings' negative behavior and write about them rather than focusing on my messed-up face and the dizzy spells. I cannot honestly say if that thought process was my heart or the tumor talking at that point. It was more like I was having conversations with myself...through Facebook posts.

Tess
July 31, 2016

Today's Tessism:
"Who cares what they think? Break the rules!"

As a (past) student of law (paralegal), I have an obsession with rules. An overwhelming need to understand them, help others understand them, and live by them.

Life has taught me that oftentimes the rule makers like to create and enforce rules while breaking the rules themselves. They make the rules up as they go along and don't always tell you what they are, so you are sure to fail at some points along the way.

But the truth is, no matter how many times you feel you are failing, and how many people may want to keep you down...there is one rule to live by that I believe will get you through:

"Do unto others as you would have them
do unto you" (Matt. 7:12).

It doesn't matter if they don't reciprocate, and it doesn't matter where you are spiritually. You can sleep at night with a clear conscience. And those who matter in your world will appreciate your kindness. If we follow but one rule in life, would we really need any others?

On the bad days, I have to remind myself that there are the rule breakers, and I must abide by the rules no matter what. And on the good days... I get to see humanity at its finest.

You see, life *is* fair. It's people who are not. When we remember this, we can forgive ourselves, and others, and focus on *living*, not being perfect.

I hope you have a fabulous day!

*****

By now, it's probably clear that I was spending a lot of time on Facebook. Where we moved, there had been only one couple we became close with, and we have appreciated them so much. Writing became my only outlet on many days; and at that point, while I was feeling my worst and not knowing what was going on with my body, I joined the "Love Your Spouse Challenge" on Facebook.

Being who I am, I "bent" the rules and used the first six days to show appreciation to friends and family. The seventh day was saved for Tony. We had seen so many obstacles in our time together, but the worst was yet to come. I'm not sure how he held it together throughout. We had literally made our vows only months before finding out how sick I really was.

*****

Tess; August 1, 2016

"And now we're standing face to face,
Isn't this world a crazy place…
Just when I thought our chance had passed,
You go and save the best for last"

Day 7 of 7, "Love Your Spouse" Challenge.

I have met the challenge from my perspective. It was important for me to give credit where it was due because recognizing the people I did for the past six days, was about some of the people who have given me hope, trust, and the renewed ability to love.

Without these experiences, I would not be able to face the "challenges" of this forever commitment.

14

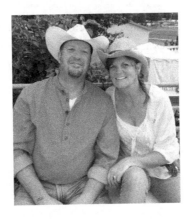

Every day, Tony takes my view of what a challenge is, wraps it in loving care…and throws it in the can! "It's only a challenge if you make it one!" And he's right.

It is not difficult to find ways to love him…the true challenge would be finding ways to stay mad.

Thank you for your smile, your touch, your support, and your love. Every day with you truly is an adventure in living!

While I was continuing to feel worse, Tony and I were dealing with life's pressures and the worst United States presidential campaign I had seen in my lifetime. My daughter was also starting to suffer. We did not know what was going on for either of us. At this point, Tony's son had successfully undergone surgery to remove the mass in his lung, and they had discovered it to be malignant. They decided not to do radiation or chemotherapy. He was doing well and starting college. He definitely deserved the title of warrior!

As for me, I realized then that I was not thinking clearly much of the time; but I dismissed it as a likely sinus infection, which often makes me feel this way. I would get them with seasonal changes, so I just took over-the-counter medications for dizziness and nausea. Still, every day I continued writing my little "blogs" on Facebook, if for no other reason than to keep the sanity that I was starting to feel like I was losing.

I was getting angry with the world and people whom I felt had wronged me or even those I love. I felt my emotions were out of control, so I kept my thoughts to myself. I told myself that it was just the stress of my relationships and life itself. I prayed for relief. For patience. For forgiveness. I thought I had never known such mercy or grace, but I realized that the Lord had been with me every step of the way. Even when I doubted and feared.

*****

Tess
August 2, 2016

Tuesday's Tessism:

If we continue thinking of people in business terms of net-gain transactions, we suffer catastrophic losses.

If we start thinking of people in terms of friends, family, and neighbors…we win at humanity.

Perspective is everything when it comes to building communities, organizations, and lives.

Tess
August 3, 2016

Today's Tessism:

When we are looking for someone to do something wrong, we *will* find it. People aren't perfect.

But when we take each other's errors and try to make the molehills into mountains, we often create a scenario that didn't need to exist.

1. Try looking for the multitude of things that person does right before pointing out their "wrong" to the world. Better yet, remember that it isn't our place to point it out to the world at all.
2. Always remember there are skeletons in our own closets, and while we're busy trying to dig up others'…someone else will gladly pull out ours.

#ThePowerOfPositiveIsUndeniable

Tess
August 6, 2016

Today's Tessism:

Everyone has a story, but the question is…will we use it to better ourselves and the world around us?

Compassion does not cost a thing, but harming others comes at a high price.

The bill may not come due today or even tomorrow, but it will come.

There is no surefire way to make it easy, but the only way to make our story honorable is to *be* honorable. There is no shortcut.

I was having to work on my own attitude. I am normally a positive person, and I love living. I don't blame God when things go wrong, but the truth is I didn't know what was wrong. I was hearing people around me suffer. Illnesses, the politics in America, and even personal relationships… People were angry! I seemed to have lost my ability to deal with people's emotions and actions, and I didn't know what to do about it. I was starting to withdraw mentally and socially.

Many times, I felt like my only "life string" to sanity was through writing blogs on Facebook. I was also starting to believe my partner did not love me anymore (I know; it's hard to imagine that after all that he had been doing for me). Furthermore, I was watching the female friends and family in my life suffering through health or relationship issues.

*****

Tess
August 7, 2016

Strong women.

Do they really exist?

I'm here to tell you, if you get out of bed every day no matter what, you're a strong woman.

Or if you set aside your own ambitions for even a moment to help someone who is struggling/suffering, you're a strong woman.

And if you speak up when others are trying to be hateful...you may feel alone, but you're a strong woman.

And if today you squared your shoulders despite the world's pressure on them...you, my friend, are going to bed tonight an incredibly, beautifully strong woman.

Tess
August 08, 2016

Too often, when we demand others to change, we are trying to change them into us.

They should think, act, react, or be the way we think they should be.

It is my (and your) responsibility to learn to accept differences and, above all, understand that there are numerous ways to accomplish one goal.

You can paint a fence a dozen different color choices, and as long as the job gets done...it's likely beautiful in any which color chosen.

Sometimes it's okay to let it be the other person's "way." What counts is that you showed teamwork and support.

In the long run, people are going to care far more about your attitude than whether you chose the "winning color."

And with the winning attitude...things will always look good on your side of the fence!

*****

Each day I was feeling worse. I was dizzy and nauseated; and though headaches weren't really common for me, I was having them every day. I knew it was time to get myself checked out. I was finally back home in New Mexico, so I went to the emergency room. I had stated that I thought I had a sinus infection, but the normal over-the-counter medication wasn't working. That maybe I needed antibiotics. One of the worst things we do to our health is trying to diagnose everything ourselves. At least I had finally made the choice to see a specialist. Afterward, I didn't do much writing for several days.

Tess
August 19, 2016

♪ This is the story of a girl... ♪

So...that little accident a few weeks ago involving my face and the sidewalk apparently turns out to have been a little nudge from my friendly guardian angel, trying to tell me I wasn't listening to previous hints that something was wrong.

After putting it off for a handful of weeks, I figured I'd better go in and see if the dizziness and headaches were due to a sinus infection, or if I had broken my nose in the fall, and it was somehow causing this.

After reviewing X-rays, the ER doctor walked back in, leaned on the table, and rested her chin on her hand. "So...did you know you have a brain tumor?" Well, I was thinking to myself that would have been the first thing I told you when I came in!

My friend Fredrica was in town, so I sent her a text; and she came to the ER immediately and waited with me.

It turned out the multiple symptoms I was trying to ignore were due to a brain tumor. I waited a few hours for an ambulance and then was transported to Lubbock, TX, for a long series of testing.

The neurosurgical team ruled out cancer in any of my other major organs (for someone with ongoing skin cancer, one of the first fears of a brain tumor is that the skin cancer has metastasized), so we will proceed with cranial surgery this coming Tuesday to remove the tumor. We will know then if the tumor is cancer. (Of course, I plan to ask since they are already there, will they just give the old face an extra nip and tuck?)

I admit I have been really dizzy and nauseated, so most technical terms the doctors use have floated right over my head. But for the most part, I feel hopeful.

There is no guarantee going in to any surgery, and this holds true for brain surgery…but I'm calm and hopeful for now. Surreal? Perhaps the Holy Spirit taking up residency in my heart.

Knowing the problem is the first step into solving it, and for me, a steady peace of mind. I have trouble with the "unknown." I need a plan to focus on.

I don't know how this will turn out, but I will face the future when it arrives. In the meantime, I will enjoy finally getting solid food tonight (yes, even hospital food). And while they're in there cutting, I've asked them to leave at least a little of the crazy that makes me Tess…

*****

At this point, humor was becoming crucial to me. I was not really clear on what was happening, so honestly, I didn't know when I was being funny or just leaning to the side of ridiculous. So I relied on others to make me laugh—anything so I could not think about the tumor or (in my mind) worse, the surgery. It didn't seem like people wanted to laugh, though.

I was admitted to the hospital in Lubbock and given a room; and as you likely know, boredom sets in quickly. Especially when you aren't able to get out and walk around. So I spent a lot of time on Facebook. In retrospect, I wonder if I should have asked the nurses or doctors for reading material on my medical condition since I simply did not ask the doctors many questions. I felt discombobulated and, truthfully, like this wasn't really happening. But as we all know, much of the information on the Internet can be misleading anyway.

I was going to rely heavily on my doctors but even more so on Tony to explain to me what the doctors were saying. Truthfully, I didn't always understand him either. I just nodded and let it bounce around inside my head until I could find something to distract me. I just wanted it all to be done. When I reached out at all, it was usually to Debi, Dana, Fredrica, and later, a new neighbor named Joyce. They have all had a different type of cancer. But the truth is I didn't reach out enough.

Tess
August 20, 2016

You know you're a redneck with a brain tumor when:

- While reading the newspaper, you make several attempts at "scrolling" through the article, only to discover that you are *not* on your phone!
- You frantically search your whole bed looking for the cell phone that is in your hand.
- Every time someone on your neurosurgeon team asks, "How ya doing?" you bust out your best Kenny Chesney dance moves (from the bed) and start singing his song "I'm Alive."
- You ask the doctor for a BOGO deal on your surgery!

Smile! Have a fantabulous day!

Nan shared a memory
August 22, 2016

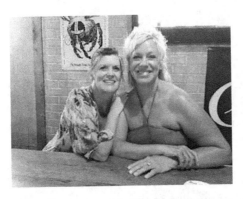

Thinking of my beautiful Tess today and lifting her into light and love before her surgery tomorrow. Some friends cross your path; and you are forever changed, laugh more, dance to life's music with wild abandon, and carry one another's tears and pain to the Keeper of joy and Healer of all.

Lubbock, Texas
August 23, 2016

Vitals and lab work and needles…oh my!
(to the tune of "Lions, Tigers & Bears")
The 4:30 a.m. view out my window. It's dark!
Just in case… I love you!

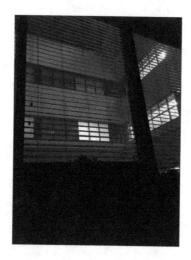

*****

I was beginning to feel emotionally numb. There had not been enough time for it to really set in, but I felt like I couldn't show my fear to anyone. Brain surgery seemed like the end. I didn't know if I was going to come out of it okay. Will I be able to see or hear? Will I be able to walk or talk or even *think* ever again? Will I still be loved? I had decided that I simply would *not* cry in front of anyone. No, I would not cry at all.

Dr. B had stopped by in the evening before the surgery to finally allow me to ask questions. This was where the first point of humor came in for me as I told the story later to friends and family. I had an offer for someone to come to the hospital and cut my long hair, so I asked Dr. B how much he would need to shave for the surgery and if I should cut it. In my memory of the situation, he shrugged and put his hands up to his ears, moving them forward toward his eyes, as he said, "If I have my way, I usually like to shave from here to here." He was shocked the next day when he came in and then said that I didn't have to cut it!

Afterward, throughout treatments, I was glad that I had and wished I had gone shorter. He told me that with the pill form of chemotherapy, patients don't always lose their hair; and if they do, it's usually only at the radiation site and may be permanent. It didn't take long for my hair to start thinning. I began to wonder if he had been trying to talk me out of having the treatments; but as much as I didn't want all the side effects that he had listed down for me, I wasn't ready to give up on living.

I didn't feel like a warrior, but I became one. It was a battle to get up in the morning and another one to lie down at night. It was another battle to attend my daily radiation appointments and another big one still to take my chemo pills. I needed sleep, but I was coming to fear it.

Tess
August 23 2016

They had me up at 4:30 a.m., drew blood again, helped me shower, and wheeled me down to holding.

Dr. B had bumped me to second string but no one knew. So here I am, back in the room waiting.

Which means it's story time!

I have a steady stream of amazing people on my medical team; and as is routine, they *all* ask, "What's your name and your birth-date?" and "Do you know what you're here for?"

So the team who will be monitoring my nervous system and blood flow stepped in, and repeating the same old questions, one spoke up, "Hi, Ms. Catt. Do you know what Dr. B is doing for you today?"

I sat up best I could, looked him in the eye, held my hands up in front of my chest, and smiled like the Cheshire Cat. "Yes! He's giving me big boobs!"

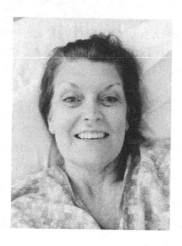

Oh my, his face went blank as he frantically searched his note-pad, and the guy next to him nearly dropped his as he turned his back to me. I could see the subtle gestures in his shoulders, of this one trying to hold back the laughter. I didn't want them to hide it. I wanted them to laugh with me. I needed some proof everything was going to be okay. I laughed sheepishly and said, "It's okay. I was teasing. I know he's removing a tumor from the center of my brain... and obviously he's going to need to give me a new sense of humor while he's in there."

*****

I genuinely did not understand the seriousness of this situation and the fact that using humor has its place. It's definitely *not* when the medical staff is checking on you.

*****

Debi
August 23, 2016

Calling all prayer warriors! My dear friend Tess will be having brain surgery today to remove a tumor. This gal brings a spark of joy and encouragement to me and so many others! Please lift her up in prayer that she can have strength, courage, comfort, and a speedy recovery. I selfishly want many more years of her friendship, so please pray for her. Dearest Tess, I wish I could be in Lubbock with you today.

Melody
August 23, 2016

Dwelling in prayer with a fellow Eagle sister and friend. Tess, we love you, and you need to know that you are riding on the strong and courageous wings of all your fellow Eagles. That's a *lot* of power! Use it well, and cling to the love as you go into battle tomorrow to kick that brain tumor's tushie!

*****

I was receiving several heartfelt messages telling me how brave I was and that everyone was praying. I didn't feel brave—I just wasn't ready to die. I was so grateful for the friends who sent messages. And I was grateful for brothers and sisters of our organization in Lubbock coming to check on me. We try so hard to be brave, but the thought of having someone cut into your brain is terrifying. You might try to give in to the fear and the feeling of loneliness, but hold on to the knowledge that you have friends and family who love you. And a (supreme) Father who will hold you in his loving arms!

I know that much of the time, I just wanted to be alone. Not so much to wallow in fear but to sleep and hopefully escape the dreaded disease in my sleep for just a little while longer. At this point, I will repeat: sending a note of encouragement is relevant to a person's recovery. This can be one of the scariest times in a person's life. And then word came.

My surgery was being rescheduled to the next day. There were twenty-four more hours to worry (or to learn not to). It was a long day of doing nothing in particular but maybe worrying, which is not the healthiest approach to surgery. It's a good time for me to suggest having a family member or friend bring in something to occupy your time: games, books, magazines, knitting, etc. Also, gather a friend or two or few family members to pray with the patient. Bring love and laughter.

The nurse gave me medication to help me sleep that night, and shortly thereafter, I did.

*****

Debi
August 24, 2016

Thinking of my sweet friend whose surgery was postponed to today. Please continue to pray for Tess. Love you, friend.

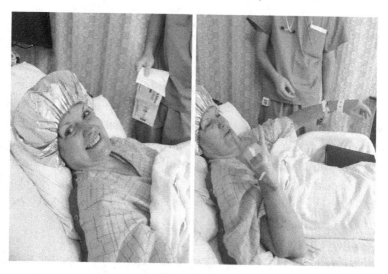

Tony added 2 new photos—feeling optimistic at UMC Outpatient Surgery.
Lubbock, Texas
August 24, 2016

This is the day for surgery. Tess is getting prepped, and we have spoken with a couple doctors so far—the team is gathering for brain tumor removal (bifrontal craniotomy).

Twenty questions or more by each doctor—an incredible coordination with each having their own specialty and responsibilities. Five visits, examinations, and sets of questions so far. Two more. Now the nurses.

They just gave her a shot, saying, "Here are your two martinis [or whatever drink of your choice] to start the process."

A kiss from Kayla and me, and she's off for an hour of more prep work. Four to six hours of surgery to follow that.

Fredrica was feeling concerned.
August 24, 2016

Okay, so *today* is the day! Please continue to pray for our friend Tess. They will be removing the tumor in her brain. Heavenly Father, please be there with the doctors, and guide them as they do this procedure on our sister. We love you, Tess, and are praying for you, Kayla and Tony.

Lep
August 24, 2016

Asking prayer for a good friend today as she faces brain surgery. This has happened very suddenly, and Tess has maintained her humor and wisdom throughout.

*****

This is not a time a person wants to necessarily be alone with their thoughts. I was and still am so grateful for the friends and family, near and far, who stood by me. While it is true to a degree when they say, "Adversity shows who your true friends are," you must know that cancer is a difficult thing to understand if you have not experienced it. So don't waste precious time being upset with people who stay back as it's their way of dealing with it. If you need them, let them know.

Tony was feeling relieved at UMC surgical ICU.
Lubbock, Texas
August 24, 2016

Gasp!

Surgery is done and went well. Tess is waking up now, within twenty minutes of completion!

Doctor B feels good about his work. Tess has been fully put back together with a handful of staples above her hairline. There will be follow-up CT scans today and another MRI tomorrow to ascertain if all of the tumor was removed. The doctor and his microscope cannot see the density differences (tumor vs. brain matter) that can be seen in the MRI—there is a possibility that he may need to go back in within the week if parts of the tumor were missed or clots form that block cerebral spinal fluid flow. He currently does not feel this will be needed—the surgery was very clean with minimal bleeding.

Tess is expected to be as fully alert as can possibly be expected within the hour.

Seems like a tremendous amount of effort and worry to lose a "quail egg" worth of weight. I would not recommend it as a weight-loss plan.

We will not know if the tumor was malignant for several days. There may be follow-up treatment of chemo or irradiation. Hopefully not needed.

I'm feeling much relieved. Thank you very much for your prayers and support.

Debi
August 24, 2016

For those of you who have been waiting to hear about Tess, I don't have much info, except I know she did come through the surgery okay, and it's a good result. Please continue to pray for her healing and strength and courage for the days ahead. Meanwhile, there's some rejoicing going on right here!

*****

Truth be told, when I woke up, I recalled that Tony was there by me; but I did not understand that the surgery had already taken place. Despite a bandage on my head, I argued that the surgery had not happened yet. I could not even remember getting prepped for it. In retrospect, maybe that was a good thing. To this day, I do not recall anything of the surgery or the prep time...only that I did not believe it had already taken place.

Tony
August 24, 2016

So as I left Tess for the evening, she was having some issues with pain medication.

Nurse entered with a breathing exercise and asked how old she was and how tall. At first, I thought the height was an unusual question for a breathing exercise. However, Tess's answer was 29 and 5'4". She had her height nearly correct, but apparently, she is much younger than I remembered.

A little later, another nurse asked if she knew her name. She immediately answered, "Kayla" (her daughter) and, stone-faced, looked directly at Kayla (who is almost 29). Later, the nurse asked where she was. No response. Nurse said, "You are at the University Medical Center." Then the nurse asked, "Do you know what town you are in?" She responded, "Town? DowntownTonyBrown!"

I laughed.

I called back a little later and talked to the new nurse on duty. She said Tess was doing great—vitals were very good. They were still trying to get her pain under control. Then she said that Tess still didn't know where she was. When that nurse had asked, Tess responded with "Hawaii!" I think she might still be upset with her boob job. LOL

*****

I will say right now: common sense tells me that I was surely just joking, but I don't really remember these conversations. And I'm sure common sense was not working at that time.

No one wants to believe their brain is not doing what it's supposed to or, worse, can create a world of its own. As time has passed, I have come to realize that memory will be one of my biggest problems. It frustrates people, so imagine how much it frustrates the person going through it. My foremost request: if you are not the patient, have patience with your loved one and yourself. If you are the patient, tell yourself that patience will be needed. Healing takes time.

For a few days after surgery, I was nauseated and dizzy, and I dealt with the pain that was normal after surgery. Somehow, my mind was still making an alternate "world," and I thought Tony had spent the night of surgery in the room with me; but I woke up in the early morning hours, throwing up and feeling pain. I don't really recall the pain these days, only that the throwing up made everything hurt. Today, I finally asked for the answer I didn't want. Tony hesitated. I don't think he wanted to upset me, but he answered. He did not recall staying overnight with me; instead, he had Kayla to care for, waiting back home.

I was determined not to cry, but it's important for me to say now that it is not a weakness to cry. Again, there is fear, pain, and a lot of unknown in this battle with cancer; and at the time, I couldn't imagine a worse illness to have. Up to this point, I really don't recall ever feeling the fear of dying; I honestly believed that I was going to live. As creative as I am, I could not imagine leaving this life before I was ready. I more so feared the disabilities I may be living with afterward. So I told myself that the only way to be strong was to just brush off the fears every time they entered my thoughts.

What this meant for me was not having much cancer conversation with anyone (not the best choice). At this point, I felt it was important to not talk about my fears because talking about them might manifest them. I often wondered if anyone had talked to me about what was going on. I did not recall anything of the surgery, and I still don't. I had come to call myself Three-minute Minnie due to the ongoing issues with short-term memory. Most people liked to tell me that it's just part of getting older. I can say this with absolute conviction at this point: I will be glad to continue doing so!

*****

Kayla
August 26, 2016

I know it's hard for you to text and see Mom, so I'll make this short.

Tonight's class was awesome and eased me in faster than I could ever imagine. The teacher is a delight and has worked with autistic students, so I am more than set to go. I love and miss you.

Tony
Lubbock, Texas
August 27, 2016

Tess just finished tearing off her occlusive bandage, getting in trouble from the nurse, and now, smiling beneath their masks. She is getting a new bandage.

Apparently she removed her own head bandages too!

She's a loose cannon!

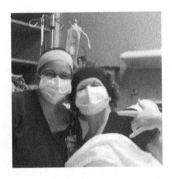

*****

I recall that I was irritated with the bandage. I genuinely felt that the medical team was trying to pull one over on me. Any other time I had surgery or a procedure, I could remember the prep time. I could not remember anything this time, and that scared me. At first, while I still had medication, I could not feel anything; so I simply did not believe they had already done surgery on me.

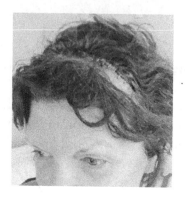

I kept replaying the theme from the *Twilight Zone* in my mind. That scared me. I needed to see for myself and also prove to myself that nothing *bad* was being hidden. It's amazing how much the brain can take and, more so, what it all can do to heal itself in these situations. I wanted to sleep, but I don't recall getting much.

Tess
Lubbock, Texas
August 27, 2016

A very nice visitor today I have not seen since high school, but he actually lives in Texas now so could come see me! I said I was his only friend who's had a lobotomy.

I have known Carlton for over thirty years. We went to high school together…and I'm blessed to say most all of us who went to Columbia Christian High School and College still touch base today! (Thankful for Facebook! Many of us have been able to reconnect and catch up with life.)

Lifelong friendships with people who live the same values, ideals, and faith that you believe in. That's amazing to me after all these years!

I've also teased with the staff about making them my home-made margaritas or Tommy's famous Chardonnay slushies, but drinking alcohol doesn't event sound appealing right now. I think you'd agree if you'd been sitting in a hospital room for about ten days watching the room spin and having to utilize those little blue plastic barf baggies. But most the time I've been in here, it's been liquid diets anyway, not solids; so it doesn't create a real big problem!

*****

Looking back on my posts, I must acknowledge that they seem silly and pointless, but writing helped me. To prove I still could. And I was blessed enough to have people in my life who just allowed me to ramble as they continued to pour out their love and support. As I am writing this "commentary" today, I fear that I have lost my creativity forever. That may seem trivial to you; but for the cancer patient, losing their strongest talent is a terrible thought. My creativity is what makes me, *me*.

Now who am I going to be?

Tess added 3 new photos.
August 28, 2016

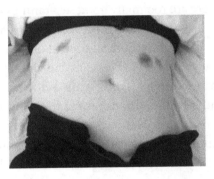

So watcha think? Zombie cheerleader for Halloween?

I'm thinking the bruising won't last for that although I get a new one in the abdomen every day via blood thinner injections.

Dr. H is keeping me today. The oncology team meets tomorrow, and he wants them to check me after they review the biopsies. I'm okay with that. I'm so dizzy I won't be fun company anyway.

Having said all this, although I won't see the pathologies until tomorrow, here is my public service announcement!

We had a friend who was keeping his skin-cancer ordeal a private affair. So only the need-to-know knew, and the general public who could have benefitted from the knowledge went unprepared. Uninformed.

This friend passed away last year from the cancer and complications. It may not have been able to be avoided for him. He did everything he could to fight it, but oftentimes it takes a preemptive strike.

Anytime a patient comes in with a brain tumor (and CT scans showed masses in the abdominal area) *and* that patient has known skin cancer, there is a concern that the skin cancer has metastasized. While this may or may not be the case for me, it has been for too many people. Skin cancer is not just an old person's disease. It can happen at any age. And it is serious. It is *not* the little or un-concerning cancer. It kills just like any other cancer, and it forever changes lives even if it does not spread to one of your major organs. Ongoing treatments are ugly and painful, and the cancer and/or treatments can be disfiguring... Not worth the so-called beauty color you get from the sun. There are too many good self-tanners out there you can get that "healthy-looking glow" from. Ask your friends, and find out who's using what. You'd be surprised to find out how many use them and how great they can look! (Please do not interpret the following line as a hint not to vote for Trump, but I do recommend avoiding the same self-tanner he did. Orange is *not* the new brown, and I hope it never will be!)

I recommend you speak to your doctor about checking your vitamin D levels if you are avoiding the sun like I have had to start doing again. You can take supplements and keep that incredible skin and just be thankful for the canvas God wrapped you in!

Be careful when choosing sunblock, and reapply often. Ask a dermatologist to recommend one.

Parents especially, don't think you are doing your toddlers any favors by getting them a cute tan to match yours. Your pride may just be setting them up for a lifetime of agony. I have known and heard of people who have died from skin cancer, ranging from 16 years old to 89 years old. This is a sometimes slow and havoc-wreaking disease.

If you have any questions, ask your doctor to refer you to a dermatologist or skin cancer specialist.

I will let you know...my skin cancer doesn't show up looking like crazy moles. It's either been scaly, rough patches that break open (often mistaken for eczema or other similar skin conditions), and sometimes it starts as a little sore that looks like a small blister or pimple but is raw and usually painful/burns to the touch and just doesn't go away. Persistent little evil skin dwellers!

I am not here to tell you how to live your lives. Just letting you know that skin cancer is more of a problem than you may realize! Suntanning is a personal choice, and as parents we love our children...we don't want to teach them to harm themselves for vanity's sake when they rely on us to keep them safe and educated! Feel free to make an impactful statement to your kids as to the importance of skin cancer awareness. When they blow it off, it's generally because we give them every reason to do so. Doesn't matter if you are dark-skinned or light. Everyone can be susceptible for different reasons.

Skin cancer is not as discriminatory as you may think! And despite what some people have said to me, it *is* serious!

Tess
August 29, 2016

♪ I'm a mustard girl in a mayo world...
(to the tune of "Barbie Girl") ♪

So...the promised update.

Hamburger for dinner with... Okay, just kidding.

The lab reports came back positive on the tumor: WHO Grade 3. Cancer.

I will be staying at the Hope House here in Lubbock for 35 to 37 days of radiation treatment and chemotherapy. (I think I will have to continue the chemotherapy for 6 to 12 months after I go home from radiation.) The masses in the liver and kidneys appear unrelated and noncancerous, so we will still not be addressing them at this time. As I hear tell... I'm in very good hands!

Prayers requested for Tony and Kayla as they go through this with me and have to carry an unexpected burden; but I know I'm loved, and they know how much I love them. And my son, Logan, so far away but deep in my heart...love and miss you!

Thank you, my friends, for the love, prayers, cards, flowers, and visits. Every time staff walks in, they say they can see how loved I am. That is the most healing power in the world, and we all need it.

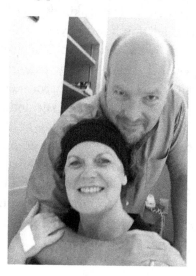

Tess
August 29, 2016

Signing out!

IVs and port are out. I get to go home for a few days!

I return in about a week to have the Frankenstein staples removed; and after that, I'll be checking in to the American Cancer Society's Hope House for about 6 to 8 weeks while having radiation and chemo treatments.

We have chosen to go with the pill form of chemo, which they can start me on right away during radiation.

I'm so happy to get to go home and be with my loves a short bit; and it sounds like my mom will be able to join me during the treatments, so I am very much counting my blessings.

I hope my friends and family know I am counting them amongst my greatest blessings! Thank you for the love, prayers, and kind words!

Always,
Tess

Tess
August 31, 2016

Oh, wow, I've lost the month of August… Where did it go?

*****

This last post in August was significant. I felt so lost then. I was so thankful for Facebook and my opportunity to write; but much of it, I didn't remember doing. I'm grateful to be able to look back and see what transpired. You might consider keeping a journal or diary yourself.

I recall feeling so very happy that I finally got to go home. I had missed my husband immensely; and my daughter had just moved to a strange state, knowing no one but Tony and myself. She and Tony had been alone together the whole time I was in the hospital. I say this because this part is imperative to those heading in to cancer care. You may feel alone, even if you are surrounded by many (and that's usually the medical team). Your loved ones are not only dealing with the worry of your diagnosis; but they also get to deal with all your following pain, the mental torment, and the physical and mental changes, all while living their daily lives.

I was afraid of losing them. *Would they be strong enough to go through this with me?* I would not be honest if I didn't say right here that it crossed my mind almost daily that I needed to just disappear. But where would I go that I would not be a burden on someone? How many people would I hurt by doing this? This is, of course, a damaging thought process, but it is an easy trap to fall into.

Tess
August 31, 2016

People keep asking, but it's hard for me to explain something I don't really understand. So I'm just putting this out there once: anaplastic astrocytoma is the diagnosis.

"Anaplastic astrocytoma is a rare malignant brain tumor. Astrocytomas are tumors that develop from certain star-shaped brain cells called astrocytes. Astrocytes and similar cells form tissue that surrounds and protects other nerve cells found within the brain and spinal cord. Collectively, these cells are known as glial cells and the tissue they form is known as glial tissue. Tumors that arise from glial tissue, including astrocytomas, are collectively referred to as gliomas. The symptoms of anaplastic astrocytomas vary depending upon the specific location and size of the tumor. The specific cause of my tumor is unknown.

Astrocytomas are classified according to a grading system developed by the World Health Organization (WHO). Astrocytomas come in four grades based upon how fast the cells are reproducing and that likelihood that they will spread (infiltrate) nearby tissue. Grades I or II astrocytomas are nonmalignant and may be referred to as low-grade. Grades III and IV astrocytomas are malignant and may be referred to as high-grade astrocytomas. Anaplastic astrocytomas are Grade III astrocytomas. Grade IV astrocytomas are known as glioblastoma multiforme. Lower-grade astrocytomas can change into higher grade astrocytomas over time."

I was given a Grade III.

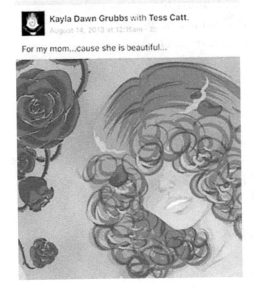

Kayla Dawn Grubbs with Tess Catt.
August 14, 2013 at 12:16am

For my mom...cause she is beautiful...

Tess
August 31, 2016

I'm home now and working on healing from the surgery so I can begin my cancer treatments.

Got up and made myself a toasted PB sandwich. Food is just not tasting right. Can't stand sweets. Ugh...

Imagine taking a bite of that peanut butter and honey. You know what taste to expect...but I swear I'm tasting that hospital casserole! *Barf!*

Baby girl is spoiling me. She gave me a nice back rub, and she won't even let me walk across the room by myself. Poor girl doesn't even realize she's turned in to me!

That big love o' mine went in to work... Thank goodness. He'd have me doing calisthenics if he could! LOL (If I could, I would too, but I'm pretty sure it'd end up on Kmart's Klassic Shoppers at some point... Sing along, "I'm so dizzy. My head is spinning...")

I just wanted y'all to know we appreciate you. Eventually this squeaky-tub-toy that keeps replaying in my brain will go away, and then I'll be back planning fun events and generally all around giving that goofy man of mine a hard time!

Until then…#LoveIsTheAnswer!

Melody to Tess
Richland, Washington
September 1, 2016

Tess, wish you were here in WA so I could pamper you! Sending you loves and prayers!

Tess
September 2, 2016

If there's only one thing I can say about prayer, it would be that it doesn't matter right now that my words and thoughts come out discombobulated. The goal is still met, and I come out feeling stronger and peaceful.

Don't knock it till ya try it! (Of course, Tony says that about his gumbo too…hmmmmmn LOL)

Have a great day!

Tess
September 2, 2016

I am convinced that a woman can be:

1. strong *and* soft
2. faithful *and* fun
3. beautiful *and* humble
4. Smart *and* Kind

Be all this…*and* still be loved *and* respected.

*Since you are already *all* this *and* more…relax. Go enjoy being everything you were designed to be and stop sweatin' the small stuff!

Tess with Tony at Rosa's Cafe
September 3, 2016

Family dinner and "catch up" time with the kiddos.

*****

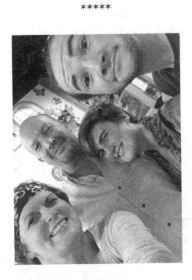

    This was my first opportunity to clean up and go out in public for a meal. I was excited but also nervous. I wanted to feel like my "old" self, but I looked in the mirror and saw the damage that the steroids were doing. Overall, I gained around thirty-five pounds in a short time; and my skin and hair became a thin, damaged mess from the chemo and radiation.) I hid the surgery site under hats and headbands daily, no matter the temperature.

    I had made it clear that I didn't really want to wear hot, uncomfortable wigs; so my daughter and I planned that if I lost all of my hair, she would "paint" henna designs on my head. It wasn't until I was well in to my radiation treatments that I realized we would not be able to do that. Although the surgical site was smooth in the beginning, my skin and the skull started to show the results of the radiation. I knew then that I was not going to be as pretty as all the cancer patients I had seen in pictures. I felt like I rather resembled a monster from the *Syfy* channel.

I never lost all of my hair; rather, it thinned and turned white, and I lost the majority of it in the radiation site. I likened it to a "halo," circling from side to side around the back of my head. The "exit point" of the radiation was my forehead; so I lost a line of hair and about half of my eyebrows, and my eyelashes were thin and brittle where they still existed. My teeth were also damaged. I had mouth sores, so I had trouble brushing really well. I also found that I was grinding my teeth and clenching my jaw in my sleep to the extent that I broke pieces off three of my back teeth. I just did my best to avoid mirrors.

*****

Tess
September 3, 2016

It's funny. I continue to write on here most every day...not really 100% sure that I'm saying what I mean to.

I've seen the storyline in many a movie, where the speaker's words aren't exactly what they intend to have come out. I don't think that's what is happening since Tony hasn't taken away my computer or phone yet! LOL.

But now we're talking something important here. *Food!*

He's making french toast from scratch, and I'm just dying to taste something good! It smells divine!

Most of the time, food is bland, like my taste buds aren't working. But sometimes tastes are completely changed... I mean, you know what dessert should taste like, but your brain keeps telling you that you're chewing on day-old dirty socks. Talk about messing with your head!

*****

I'll add right here that I don't really know what day-old dirty socks taste like; but it was what came to mind when I would eat.

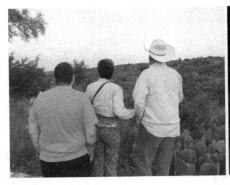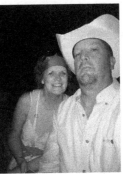

Tess
September 4, 2016

Night flight of the bats
Carlsbad Caverns, New Mexico

My husband tried to get me out of the house often. He was worried that I would just lie there and give up on life. It didn't do any good to tell him when I didn't feel well. Just as well since I wanted to share our little corner of the world with my daughter and her friend who was visiting from Wisconsin.

*****

Tess
September 5, 2016

He's making sure we're well taken care of Mom...
Fresh-grilled burger, homemade coleslaw from fresh cabbage (said to have anti-cancer fighting properties and good stuff for healing since the surgery), and veggies from our own garden!

*****

It really didn't matter to me what he gave me to eat since things simply didn't taste like they were supposed to. I was grateful that he was there and that he loves cooking. I was also letting myself worry about him and my daughter instead of resting.

While I was indeed starting to eat again, it seemed then that I was heavy on steroids to keep down the edema after surgery, so I couldn't stop eating. My weight was soaring! I had a nurse and physical therapist who came in to my home a few days a week. This was mostly precautionary because many patients who come out of brain surgery have difficulty with physical activity and talking, and some even suffer strokes.

I am going to stop here for a moment to interject again on the importance of being positive, especially for friends and caregivers. It is difficult and frightening as a patient goes through treatments and recovery from a major surgery, constantly hearing stories of others' experiences with cancer ending in death. While it is truly a blessing that your family member had two to five happy years before passing, a current patient needs to focus on healing—being healthy and positive and possibly even having something to look forward to.

For a few people, it might serve to motivate; but for others, it's a catapult to fear and worry. Be sure you know your patient well before sharing stories of fellow cancer patients.

Tess
September 6, 2016

Physical therapist just left. I feel very blessed to have a medical team that comes to my home until I check in to the American Cancer Society (ACS) Hope Lodge, back in Lubbock, next week... I think it makes it easier on everyone. The PT was thrilled with Tony's choice of power food for my dinner last night (a bit of fatty beef and fresh cabbage coleslaw, apparently two vital foods for healing the brain). And today's after-lunch snack consists of Greek yogurt, fruits and nuts, and a potassium-rich banana. I'm pretty sure this will not be a weight-loss experience for me. Between Tony's successful meals and the steroids, the desire to eat again has been kick-started...and now I just feel like I'm eating nonstop! LOL.

I did, however, have a successful walk to the mailbox and back! Woo-hoo! I'll be ready for that *Iron Man* marathon in no time!

Okay, on to the important stuff! My most sincere thank-you to friends and family who have taken time to leave or mail a note(s); thank you for the flowers and gifts and meaningful little texts... You may never know for sure the difference it makes in one's attitude and willpower, but believe me when I say it matters!

*****

After my brain surgery, I was determined to walk every day and get back to exercising, definitely not understanding the reality. The doctor approved, but I had to be assisted by my PT and nurse; and he emphasized the statement, "as long as your body can handle it." Turns out, it was harder than I expected. A walk to the end of block required another person with me at all times. One block was exhausting and sometimes painful, and it made me feel older than my age. It was easy to fall since I could not keep the dizziness at bay. I was scared that I would never be "normal" again.

To be clear, I'm not really the type of lady everyone considers "normal." I talk excessively, I have my fair share of insecurities, and I tend to view things differently than the crowd. On the good side of all that, I was very creative and loved using that ability at every given opportunity. At this point, I would have given anything to be the old me; but over time, changes started showing.

My husband stated more than once that I had changed; but to me, I liked some of the changes. I could see that I was not worrying so much about what people thought of me or what I had to say. He never really told me what it was that he thought had changed about me, but I started realizing that my memory (mostly short term) was affected and that I could no longer multitask. This meant that people had to give me directions or instructions one piece at a time.

I was so embarrassed. I found myself wondering often if he was wishing that I hadn't made it through the surgery, or if he wished he had chosen someone else over me. I also discovered that if I was dreaming, I no longer remembered it, at least as a dream. Most often, it became my reality.

At this point, I was struggling. Overall, I was on the steroids for about four months, trying to ensure that I did not have the worrisome issues, like edema that follows brain surgery and treatments. I will be completely honest and say that treatments have many side effects; but for me, I wasn't thinking about those side effects (until I was deep into them). I only thought that I was not ready to die a slow and miserable death from brain cancer, much less leave my family behind. And the mental anguish had begun setting in.

Tess
September 6, 2016

I think I will sleep well tonight. I'm simply too tired not to.

Truth is… I have worried. I have been angry, and I feel so small in this great, big world.

I am so angry that my loved ones have to go through this and that I cannot make everything right in this world for them.

People chose to love me and have faith in me, and I feel like I'm failing them big time. So much to do but I'm so tired all the time.

This isn't how it is supposed to be We are supposed to be making the world a better place, not just sitting here waiting for me to get better.

It doesn't seem real. What a strange place for me to be caught in—no control over anything, when all I've ever really thought I've been in this world…is a fixer.

And I don't know how to fix my broken self so that I can just keep on fixing.

I'm sorry. I want to be brave and be strong. And I look into the eyes of people I love and hurt that I am causing them sadness and hardship. When all I want to bring them is love. And peace.

Time to sleep. I'm simply too tired not to.

*****

I was scheduled the next day to have my staples taken out, and that meant another two-hour trip to Lubbock. I had to keep reminding myself that folks who live in this little oil-field town in New Mexico repeatedly stated to get important medical care out of town. I couldn't imagine this not falling into that category; but the two-hour drive was impossible for me at that point, which meant that Tony had to take yet another day off from work to drive me.

*****

Tess
September 7, 2016

Staples out. Now radiation and chemo all set up.

He's treating me to Five Guys burgers now! I'm a "hungry hungry hippo!"

*****

I was truly blessed. I could have wallowed in the worry and fears; but I was trying to make the best out of a difficult, if not bad, situation. As I look back, the memories of those hardships have already started fading; but more importantly, I have been able to recognize all of the good that came out of this. Cancer is never good, but God certainly has granted me mercy and has been patient and brought many wonderful new people in to my life. I cannot begin to imagine this journey without my family and friends. I also cannot imagine having to go through this again!

Tess
September 7, 2016

Holy cow!

Did I not tell y'all to warn me before I let Tony at me again (after the "foot-carving for a little sliver" incident last year?)

During my shower, I discovered two staples the nurse missed... Nope, Tess couldn't wait to go see a doc tomorrow. Had to have Tony pull them out tonight.

I'm pretty sure there isn't an enemy alive that could be meaner to me than I am myself!

Not to worry. I'm sure by tomorrow afternoon, I will have found another way to punish myself again!

*****

At this point, what I was going to go through was most likely going to feel like an emotional roller-coaster, and I had not even started treatments yet! I don't know about others' experience; but I was really feeling isolated, scared, and absolutely not ready to face everything. Still, I didn't talk about it. I did not want to add any burden onto my loved ones. So I put on my tough face every day and tried to pretend it did not hurt my feelings when my partner didn't seem to understand what I was going through.

In my mind, I thought, *If he's already showing signs of being frustrated with me at this point, how was it going to be a few months from now? A year from now? Two years?* (I will state here for the record that as I am writing this, it has been a bit more than two years after the surgery, and my guy stuck through all of this. He's still here, still making me laugh, and still showing me his love and support!)

*****

Tess
September 8, 2016

Beautiful day!

Finished with physical therapist; then my daughter took a walk around the block with me.

Followed up with my Herbalife shake, blended with fresh blueberries, banana, strawberries, and a dash of Greek yogurt… Yummy!

Tess
September 8, 2016

An update for those trying to keep up:

I will go back in next week for all my preliminaries to treatments; and then thanks to the American Cancer Society, I have a room near the treatment facility in Lubbock, where three very lovely ladies in my life will each take a turn spending some time with me as my support system.

With the help of the South Plains (Lubbock) Fraternal Order of Eagles Auxiliary, and Aerie members Lonnie and Jerry and Nancy, my mother is able to fly in and spend a week or so with me toward the end (late October or early November).

And our sweet friend Nan will be coming to spend some time in early October, which I know will keep me in constant smiles. My daughter, Kayla, will fill in the "blank" times.

How can anyone be afraid with so much love and goodness in their corner?

I, for one, am starting to feel excited about all the opportunities that can arise from what might sometimes feel like a dark situation.

Please keep all these beautiful people in your prayers, and continued blessings for my Tony and Kayla for standing through the struggle right by my side every step of the way!

It's a great day to have a great day!

Tess
September 8, 2016

Today was a good day. Not because I was short on pain or dizziness/nausea (that has been in fruitful abundance today). But because the entire medical team that works with me likes to remind me how loved they can see I am and how I am actually doing really well under my circumstances.

In truth, it's hard to believe I really have the condition they say or that they GPS'd their way through my brain to remove a complex tumor. I sort of expect to just wake up each morning and find it was just a dream. Too much Syfy channel?

But truth is…there is one thing I know to be real in all of this, and that is the *love* of good people in this world.

Trust me on this one, my friends…*never* sell yourself short! Every day it is within your power to make a difference. And if you might doubt that, just know that tonight I was full-on belly laughing with Tony and Kayla. Despite a more-than-just-a-little discomfort kind of day, I felt the bigger picture in my life. And *you* have been a part of that. How does a girl get so lucky?!

Thank you for being you and sharing that hope, faith, and love with me.

Tess
September 11, 2016

When I first heard Disturbed's remake of "The Sound of Silence," it reached deep down in my soul and grabbed ahold of my heart.

Today I heard it along with pictures that grabbed me by the throat to shake me awake.

Now is not the time to attack fellow citizens verbally or otherwise. And shame on the so-called leaders on every level who think it is okay to verbally blast others and encourage others to do so. That is not leadership. That is a selfish display of the false pedestal you put yourselves on.

It takes a lot less effort to bite down a bit on one's tongue and offer love and encouragement as opposed to putting others down to make yourself feel good.

Shame on you for thinking you could be a good leader for me. Shame on me for allowing it to get this far. Shame on fellow Americans who think it is ever at any time okay to attack your brother and sister instead of lifting him/her up. It amazes me that we think we can persuade others to see our view by shoving it down their throats with hate and violence.

It is your choice whether to believe in any super deity/religion and most certainly your freedom (not right; just freedom) to voice your opinion against mine…but we got off track.

To clarify…opinion is only that. It is not necessarily fact, truth, or honorable just to open your mouth to push your point. Strength and courage isn't shooting off our mouths in attack of another.

Courage is showing love to someone who is down.

Courage is biting your tongue when you want to say something mean.

Courage is fighting a fair and honest battle for those who cannot do it on their own.

Courage is showing *love* when surrounded by hate.

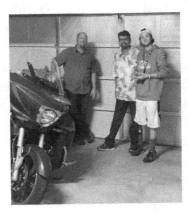

Tess Catt
September 21, 2016

The boys all together again and Tony's famous barbecue… What more could a girl ask for?

Tess Catt
September 23, 2016

While those crazy men are fighting bad weather on motorcycles, headed for Four Corners Regional Conference, Kayla is spoiling me with a mani/pedi, and I'm working on garage crafts. I feel a bit bad for her, stuck taking care of me. Anyone who knows me knows how quickly I go stir-crazy.

And just for you, Babe, I'm listening to Kid Rock's cover of "Turn the Page." Be safe. Be happy. Be #EagleStrong

Tess Catt
September 23, 2016

As "corny" as it may sound, counting blessings is important. It is relevant.

Under my current circumstances, I'm not supposed to get caught up in the little things like weight gain, hair loss, or the swelling in my face/neck. That comes down to vanity...right?

But we spend our lives being judged. For our looks. Our actions. Our beliefs.

We're harder on ourselves than anyone else could ever be.

And I'm tired. Sometimes I can't stomach looking in the mirror, and I feel weak that my daughter has to let me hold her arm as we walk around the block. I want to be strong.

This isn't intended to be a complaint so much as an acknowledgment...that in my fatigue, I am so grateful that I have blessings to count. I *need* to count my blessings, and thankfully, there are so many I'd likely fall asleep before I can finish.

It's also important for me to remind you that you are a blessing. Maybe mine, maybe for others...but you are relevant. You give strength when you may not even realize it.

I know I'm not perfect, but I do believe in the perfection of love and what we have to offer each other. And some days, that's all I think I have to hold on to.

So what I'm saying is...you please hold onto that too. Don't let fears or politics or negative people stop you from believing in *you* and what you are capable of!

You've already come this far. *Don't* stop now!

Tess Catt
September 24, 2016

Time to get this party started!
Let your inner beauty bloom this beautiful Saturday morning…
by helping someone else get their bloom on!

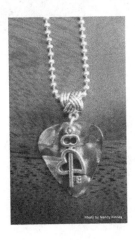

Nancy shared a photo to your Timeline.
September 24, 2016

I've always called this "the key to your heart." You have the hearts of many of us here. I am putting together your care package very, very soon. Had to get a couple things meant especially for you. You are loved.

Tess
September 25, 2016

Got the aging patina done. Now need to step away and make myself take a nap while it dries.
I'm excited to get the beautiful wooden desktop stained and finished that Tony hand built.

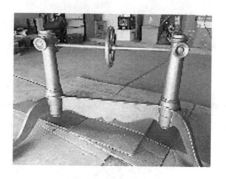

Tess
September 25, 2016

Okay…break from garage crafts for this very important update! HAPPY BIRTHDAY TO THE MOSTEST AWESOMEST MAMA—our angel on earth, the wind beneath my wings!

Tess
September 25, 2016

Western Bacon Burger and fried zuccinni. Thank heaven for the little things.

(But Kayla kept trying to take my burger away so I wouldn't overstuff myself and be miserable. Now *that's* not a little thing! LOL.)

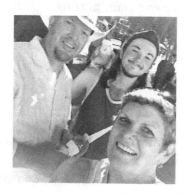

Tess
September 26, 2016

Good morning! I hope you have been able to start your day so far with laughter and sunshine!

Today was my last in-home care visit from my nurses and PT. I've grown fond of them in a short time, so I will miss them (even though they all made sure I had their numbers to text them! Oops!). But tomorrow is the big day. Scheduled to start the radiation and chemo and move into the ACS Hope House.

Obviously a little nervous about it all but anxious to get it started...and completed! LOL

However, today's nonstop smile is brought to you by the Big Guy, who is on his way home now. Can't wait to see his perfect smile!

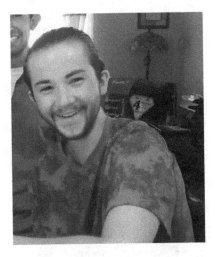

Tess
September 26, 2016

Well, if we're going to do it in the Brown household, we're going to do it up big!

Just got home from Jesse's follow-up from the lung surgery in July.

He's doing awesome but has decisions to make regarding his treatments.

Sarcoma is one of the cancers that metastasize; the cells will hide away in the various spots and may eventually resurface. In Jesse's case, it resurfaced in his lung. As I understand it, the surgeon did a good job of removing the affected area. But now Jesse heads in for PET and bone scans to try and find any lurking little demons before choosing and beginning his plan of defense. A brave 19-year-old indeed.

In case I don't say it enough... Thank you, Tony, for being our *rock*!

Janet to Tess
September 27, 2016

Thinking of you today.

*****

Some days were worse than others; but then notes, calls, cards, etc., would come in and bring a smile back to my face through any discomfort. It means the world to know that there are people out there cheering you on in the battle. You can face another day, another needle, another test, and soon after, the treatments.

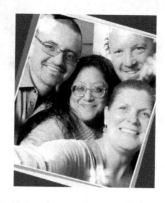

Fredrica
Seminole, Texas
September 27, 2016

So last year this crazy couple came into our lives, and we fell in love with their souls! People talk about soul mates I believe in "soul besties." So a few months ago, I get this call from my friend Tess. "Hey, girlfriend, just wanted to let you know I'm in the ER, and they are sending me to Lubbock. They found a mass in my brain." Trying to be strong for her, I rushed to be by her side and to see what I could do. They later removed her tumor, and today she starts her radiation and chemo journey. I will never understand why there is cancer or why it chooses the people it does; but I do know that we have a powerful God, and he is going to get my friend Tess through this. Please keep her and her lil' family in your prayers as they go through this not only with her, but with Tony's son as well, who is fighting his own cancer battle. My dearest Tess, you, my dear, are *not* alone! God will carry you through it all. I love you, I love you, I love you!

Nan added 3 new photos—with Tess.
September 27, 2016

Cancer picked the wrong opponent with my beautiful friend, Tess. Her positive attitude doesn't back down when fear throws a pass her way. She's the quarterback of comebacks, and she throws touchdowns to every play of hope! Brain cancer hasn't tackled her, can't keep up with her on the field of life, and she is heading for the touchdown of recovery. I have the gift of flying to be with her in TX next week for a few days as she begins a month-long radiation and chemo treatment. Brain cancer doesn't know that all those nights of dancing that we shared have given her the fitness to leave it in her dust on the 40-yard line... No field goal, no tie, no overtime... She's running for a Super Bowl kind of touchdown and victory!

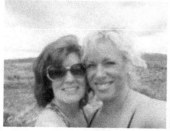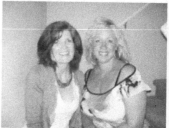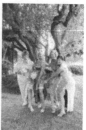

Tess
September 27, 2016

Many of you have seen the beautiful note on my Facebook wall from the mysterious Nan, who will be coming to spend a few days with me next week at the Lodge. (The Hope Lodge, overseen and paid by the American Cancer Society, is similar to the Ronald McDonald house but is a place for adults who are specifically receiving cancer treatments and is set up for one person to stay with us as a "caregiver." As a brain surgery/cancer patient, I am not allowed to stay alone due to all the risks.)

This is my way of sharing a piece of our Nan with you so you cannot only know the joy she is, but feel free to envy my position a wee bit. After all, if you're going to do something silly like get brain cancer…you should be smart enough to ensure you've got the best people in your corner!

("Kitchen Talks" by Nan Riddle can be found on YouTube.)

Tess
September 27, 2016

Oy vey!
Sadly, I've been rescheduled. Radiation was set to start. We drove the two hours, but the chemo prescription did not arrive yet. Radiation and chemo docs agree that they want both treatments to start at the same time…so tentatively scheduled to return to Lubbock on Sunday for check-in to Hope Lodge, and hopefully start treatments Monday or Tuesday. *sigh*

It seems to me I'm going to have to suck it up and spend the next week finding creative ways to occupy myself! Hopefully, it doesn't involve more eating! LOL

Fredrica
Seminole, Texas
September 28, 2016

So we've been going through so many trials in our lives lately, but we have *never* lost sight of who our God is and just how good he is! And today my love sent me this picture he took. God's soldier protecting us!

GOD IS GOOD ALL THE TIME!
ALL THE TIME GOD IS GOOD!

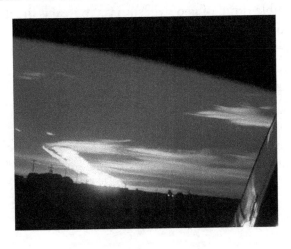

Tess
September 28, 2016

I'm so happy! Today is a good morning. I am up and around, feeling free of both pain and dizziness this morning! Amazing! (So much so, I treated myself to a coffee this morning, a luxury for me right now!)

Yummy Kona coffee, a courtesy of the beautiful Bambi; and the Cup-O-Luv, courtesy of the kindhearted Kim; and *glorious sunshine*, courtesy of our heavenly Father! A bit of extra sleep tucked sweetly in, courtesy of that handsome cowboy known as Downtown Tony Brown.

It has totally put me in the mood to run a marathon! (But I will be good and start off with my garage projects and a bit of CCR playing on the radio!)

My wish for you today is multiple reasons to smile…and an opportunity to serve someone who can never give you anything back but gratitude!

Much love!

Tess
September 28, 2016

It's always a great day to be kind. Be patient, and be smart!
The Bible is full of goodwill stories…but so is life if we watch!
It's a beautiful day to be alive!

Tess
September 28, 2016

Daughter approved, date ready.
Dinner and a movie :)
(I think I started a wee bit early in my enthusiasm! LOL)

Heavenly Father,
May every cancerous
cell be cast out and
replaced with a good
one. May every spot
of this deadly cell be
wiped out by Your
powerful hands.
Amen.

Bill
September 28, 2016

Tess.

Tess
September 29, 2016

Easy, breezy CoverGirl kind of day! Okay...mind you, I'm not looking CoverGirl; but Kay and I walked to Starbucks on this cool, windy September morning. Forewarning to those considering a sort-of-lobotomy, make a note in your phone that Frappuccino brain freezes suck...and if you don't leave yourself some kind of note, you'll forget and be right back there a few days later trying to do it again! A good day, but we're missing our coffee cohort Tommy O!

Tess
September 29, 2016

Joanne—thank you for the reminder of this awesome song ("Fight Song" by Rachel Platten).
I'm at the beginning, and feel there's going to be mornings that I'm going to want to set this as my wake-up alarm.

In reality, everyone has a battle they face at some point, and what we want to walk away from all this with is that we're stronger than we think…but thankfully don't have to do it alone.

This is… "Take back my life song!"

Debi
September 29, 2016

Add this one to *your* playlist, Tess! I especially love the line "All of a sudden I am unaware of these afflictions eclipsed by glory." ("How He Loves Us" by David Crowder Band)

*****

Don't forget to check out music therapy while on your journey. Music can aid with laughter, smiles, and yes, even getting the tears out. Some songs can specifically give you courage and strength.

Tess
September 29, 2016

Every day we are given numerous opportunities to make our own personal choices.

Sometimes, things happen whether we choose or not, but there is never a time we aren't given the chance to choose our (mental/spiritual) reaction.

In truth, I know I'd rather have to make attitude choices about something like someone talking behind my back, than minute-by-minute attitude choices regarding my health/treatments/discomfort…but *life happens*; and what we learn is that in the end, whatever the situation, *you stand.*

And thankfully fellow human beings on this journey called *life*, step up and sometimes even hold you up in the stand. (See the song by Rascal Flatts, "Stand.")

Tess shared a memory.
September 30, 2016

Some days I crack myself up. Some days I just scare myself!

Tess
Washington
September 30, 2013

No sleeping when you have a flold (flu/cold); at least I didn't catch a clu! Bwahahaha! Note to self: chill on the NyQuil.

*****

I spent many days and nights being afraid. There are no promises, and if I'm going to be honest, it wasn't death I feared (although I do fear pain a bit). It was more so that I needed to make sure that my children were set if I were to leave this physical life. My son is in the military. He's a smart young man and is making his way. But my daughter, for all her talent and smarts, simply was having trouble facing life with her disabilities. I needed to know that I had the time to help her get on the right footing. Or that God grants her the right people to help her stand.

Rebecca is feeling inspired.
September 30, 2016

What an eye-opener so early this morning! Thanks again to you, Tess, for always sharing with us. I must confess it was the "cat puke" blog that got me and drew me in… Ugh, can't handle that very well. This blog by Dawn D is so *spot on*! Wouldn't this world be so wonderful if we would each try to follow the guidance set forth for us so many years ago! I try to find the good and to encourage and build up my sisters and brothers. I must admit that it has recently been very difficult to overlook some things and try this rework method. I must now try even harder.

Thanks again so very much for sharing this.

Teresa updated her cover photo.
September 30, 2016

*****

This picture wasn't about taking a ride off a cliff. Instead, it's about having people you care about stay by your side in this ride called life.

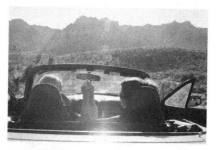

Thelma & Louise forever

*****

Alvin to Tess
Spokane, Washington
September 30, 2016

Pleased to meet you. Let's chat and get to know each other.

Laura
September 30, 2016

For you, Sweetie. Lots of prayers to you.

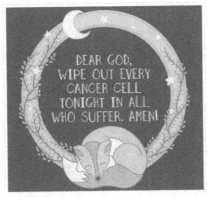

DEAR GOD,
WIPE OUT EVERY
CANCER CELL
TONIGHT IN ALL
WHO SUFFER. AMEN!

Stop cancer. Start praying. Visit ePrayCancer.com

Terry
September 30, 2016

"My Hero of the Month, October, 2016"—Tess Catt.

A mom, a friend, a love, a confidant, a fighter. She took a tumble (face-plant), and after days and days of discomfort, she went to the doctor. The tests revealed a brain tumor. The surgery results: a malignancy. While many would cower, she rose to meet her opponent with strength and courage!

Her words: "Trust me on this one, my friends...*never* sell yourself short! Every day it is within your power to make a difference. And if you might doubt that, just know that tonight I was full-on belly-laughing with Tony and Kayla. Despite a more-than-just-a-little-discomfort kind of day, I felt the bigger picture in my life. And *you* have been a part of that."

Her positive nature, strength, courage, genuineness, love, and laughter make her "My Hero of the Month, October, 2016"—Tess Catt.

Tess
September 30, 2016

Uh-oh, run for the hills… The docs warned Tony and I that I might be moody and irritable!

I really don't mind getting older. There are lots of benefits. But one of them may not be for some of the young hairstylists. Bless their hearts. If you're 50 and rising, apparently, they don't think you care about style (or that you realize there is more than one for your age).

Sweet young thing, may I just say… I'm not fond of bowl cuts! I didn't particularly want the one-size-fits-all haircut for mature women. Doggonit, I like being me, not Mrs. Cleaver!

Serious mom-haircut affliction going on here!

Deep breath…a good night's sleep, and I will talk Tony into taking the clippers to it in the morning.

Just about anything has got to look better than the accidentally asymmetrical bowl cut!

On the bright side, they tell me I'm going to lose it all anyway. But I'll be darned if I'm going to walk around leaning my head to one side until that happens!

*****

It's so funny to me that I would care about the haircut. I mean, odds are I'm going to lose the hair, anyway. Life is definitely full of the lessons, and where they come from can be very surprising.

*****

Tess
September 30, 2016

Next to inspiring people, it's what he does best. Well...almost. Chicken cashew stir-fry, straight off the grill! And he even used veggies from our garden, like hot red peppers, onions, and carrots.

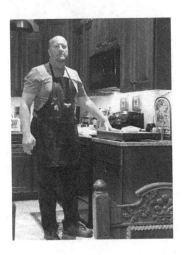

Tess
October 1, 2016

My happy place.
Where it doesn't matter that my hands are shaky,
My memory is faulty,
And I can't fit in my cutest outfit.
This is where our ideas come to life!
*Desk/top for metal antique drawing table base.

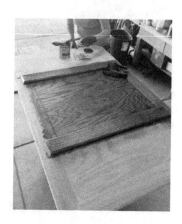

Tess
October 1, 2016

When you let your man cut your hair.
The barber of Seville took his share!
I took some regular scissors to it and fine-tuned it a bit...
Will show you the finale after I get cleaned up!
Scary... I know! LOL

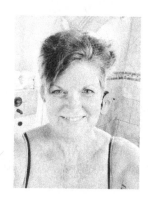

Tess
October 2, 2016

When negativity hits, you feel like judging or that you are being judged… Just remember.

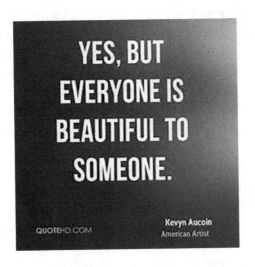

Tess
October 3, 2016

Top of the morning to you, you glorious Monday maniacs!
May your day be productive, your heart be full, and your attitude appropriately crazy!
The rest of the "normals" will catch up shortly!

*****

Are you feeling the roller-coaster ride yet? Emotions go everywhere, including the dark places—places you don't want to know exist. And then there were times when I was mentally existing in another world. My mind was busy making up all kinds of alternative realities, and I was not aware that the things I was saying weren't real.

I could no longer tell the difference between reality and the dreams I couldn't remember having.

Tess
October 3, 2016

I'm going to have to figure out some silent hobbies to take up during all these nights of insomnia! Not so much thinking sudoku.

Now it's time to wake up the family and prepare to head back to Lubbock. Another round of doc appointments today and then treatments expected to begin this week.

Kayla will be with me at the ACS Hope Lodge until Wednesday. Then I have our effervescent Nan all to myself (well, okay, I'll share her with the other patients/visitors). And then we'll round out October with my beautiful mother!

In all honesty, I'm not excited about this adventure. It's one of those times when you're anxious to get it started so you can get it over with… But I'm starting my day with the prayer that we all have the strength and love to meet our "hardships" head-on and heart full. That we can rise to our challenges together and meet them with grace, dignity, and honor.

I'm tired and a bit scared, but I promise this one thing to myself and loved ones… I will do my best to see the good in every day that follows!

Thank you for allowing me your friendship, love, and insight along this journey. I couldn't do it without you!

*****

I have to laugh when I see the comment about Sudoku. At an appointment in mid-2019, I was discussing my memory issues with my oncologist. He asked if I played "any of those phone games." I replied that I had played a few but don't usually do so. He then suggested I play Sudoku. I laughed at that one. I told him, "I wasn't any good at that game before all this, so unless the surgeon did something magical while inside my head, I'm not thinking I'll start now!" Thankfully, my oncologist was/is patient!

*****

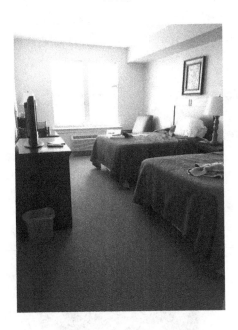

Tess
October 3, 2016

Kayla and I are settled in to my room at the ACS's Hope Lodge. Putting away the way too many clothes I always bring on trips! LOL

A true blessing that allows me to take my daily treatments without having to drive two hours each way.

Tonight we are headed down to the common dining area to be served dinner by a local sorority from Texas Tech University. Should be fun and hopefully a good experience for Kayla to mingle.

I'm pretty sure I'll lose her to the library before dinner even gets served! LOL

Tess
October 3, 2016

Quote of the day: "Love is the ability and willingness to allow those that you care for to be what they choose for themselves without any insistence that they satisfy you" (Wayne Dyer).

Terry to Tess
October 5, 2016

Go, go, go, Hero!

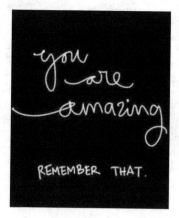

Tess
October 5, 2016 at 12:00 p.m.

Today is a good day, Terry! My labs all came back great, and after completion of chemo education… I have pills in hand! Should start both radiation and chemo by next Monday. So tonight, volunteers from a local church are serving up Mexican casserole… I'm totally planning to pig out! LOL. Have a wonderful day, my dear!

Tess
October 4, 2016

You never really recognize how "automated" you have become until your world changes.

"Hi! How are you doing?" It's well intended, but I say it often before I even realize what has come out of my mouth.

In a "house" full of sick people, it's a tough greeting, though. I don't want to answer "honestly" knowing that they are as miserable, if not worse than I am.

And yet here, we all have something in common, so we can let down our guard. No need to feel insecure about the distorted/swollen face. Don't have to hide the shaky hands, or feel ashamed that my daughter is my "anchor" keeping me from stumbling over my "jelly legs."

We can all breathe easy and just smile at each other.

Last night, while I rested after dinner, Kayla went back down to the dining room; and there she met and visited with John and Beverly. We ran into them this morning on our way out for my walk, and they were genuinely pleased that Kayla remembered their names. They were cheerful and welcoming, having been here awhile already for John's treatments.

Honestly, it's a strange thought to know you fit in, in a small "world" of people who are sick. But what we can come away from this with is recognizing that we are all in this world together; and while we have a tendency to separate our world into convenient little niches, we are all united by our humanity...and we maintain that unity through love.

Don't get me wrong. Love doesn't mean you particularly have to like me as a person or hang out like best friends. Love is simply treating others with kindness. Respect. Dignity.

You know...the kind of treatment we demand of others toward ourselves.

Yes, indeed. It is the season of change, and I intend to welcome it no matter how much it may scare me or how I may fear the unknown.

Just remember...your spouse/partner, your children, your friends, and even your job were at one time the unknown.

In fact, each of us at some point have been someone's "unknown."

And we have the power within us to help others lose their fear of that unknown...by using the love already within us!

Tess
October 5, 2016

YouTube song—"Beautiful Day" by Jamie Grace.

Good morning, family and friends!

Here's my smile for you today...and my most sincere thank-you for choosing to be beside me in spirit on this path.

Fear tries to be our exclusive partner on our individual journeys, but *love* ensures we are surrounded with goodness... No room for *fear*!

Let's get this show on the road!

Back-to-back appointments this morning, including more chemo education. Then our girl Nan arrives this afternoon to keep my head on straight for the next few days...

How does a girl have it so good?

Why, *you*, of course!

See y'all on the flip side of this *beautiful* day!

Rebecca
October 5, 2016

"Amazing Grace" always seems to touch the soul, and I had always loved it played on bagpipes. However, there is nothing as beautifully haunting as the version by David Doring on the pan flute with the beautiful natural scenery as a backdrop. It can calm and soothe even on the worst of days. Just think what it does on a great day. Tess, Penny, Cathy, Pat, Janet, JanetJ, Pat, Mary, Pat, Beverly, Kim, Tony, Diana, Jean, Joyce, Kathy, Lisa.

Tess
October 5, 2016

Look! It's a beautiful Florida mermaid!
(Actually, Nan is originally from Texas, so she's feeling right at home!) My days just got sunnier!

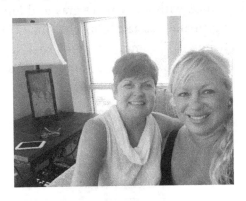

Nan
October 5, 2016 at 2:47 p.m.

I am smiling as big as TX here with my beautiful Tess at the American Cancer Society Hope Lodge! She is one amazing woman, and I am one lucky friend! Just to warn you, we will be planning her makeover after her treatments and her victory party!

Tess
October 5, 2016
Today I received a lovely balloon bouquet from Terry and Phil. It brightens up our room!
Now Nan and I are out walking the Texas Tech Campus...lots of young-uns here!

Tess
October 5, 2016

I'm going to bed very happy and exhausted!

Had a fun and active day with Nan, got to make new friends from the group of volunteers from the local Church of Christ who cooked up and served a wonderful dinner for the patients and care-givers, met some of my fellow patients staying at the lodge...and *finally* have my start date for radiation and chemo treatments to start (again)...da-da-da-daaaa...*tomorrow*!

"When I'm stuck with a day that's gray and lonely, I just stick out my chin and grin and saaaaay, 'Oh! The sun'll come out tomorrow, so ya gotta hang on 'til tomorrow, come what may!'

Tomorrow! Tomorrow! I love ya tomorrow! You're only a day away!"

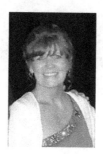

Nan
October 6, 2016

Today she didn't have to be strong, in charge, powerful, or a conqueror. Today she just had to show up. And some days that's the most important thing to do. Show up.

#firstradiation&chemoDONE.

October 6, 2016 at 1:47 p.m.

Showing up was easier with someone holding my hand!

Tess
October 6, 2016

First day of radiation successfully behind me. My chemo is not the traditional intravenous, but I am on a pill form, which allows me to be on the chemo treatments while doing the radiation treatments; and I will take my first one tonight before bed.

I will continue the radiation and chemo five days a week (weekends off) for about seven weeks; then we will determine the next step from there.

Our sweet Nan was by my side all day, with smiles and silly sayings to keep my humor up.

It's been most humorous when she says things like, "Oh, I can't believe I just asked you to help me remember," and taking me on a beautiful evening walk while leaving me in charge of the direction. Hahahahaha! Yes, we did feel a wee lost for a bit.

*****

It's true. Some days were actually funny! Amazing. Beautiful. Strengthening. I was slowly learning that it is within each of us to make a positive out of the negative. It is difficult to believe that I had the internal keys to get this old engine shining brightly every day. Maybe I was not running on high-performance level yet, but my attitude was my choice. And yes, I do understand that it's easier said than done.

Tess
October 7, 2016

As I lay down on the slab to get my head "pinned" to the table, the radio started.

You know it's a "here's your sign" moment when "Another One Bites the Dust" comes on first thing. Now, how it happened exactly: I stepped in the room, jumped up onto the metal "bed"; and as the two techs stood conversing in the corner, I started looking up at the ceiling (speakers) and raised an eyebrow, looking around the room. The techs caught my behavior; and one came over, resting his hand gently on my shoulder. "Is there anything I can do for you? Do you need anything?" And I smiled a crazy half-grin and replied, "Did you guys pick this song just for me?" He looked mortified, but I laughed and said, "No, no…it's referring to the cancer cells and my radiation!"

Yeah, the radiation techs and I had a good laugh over that one!

*****

I lived each moment waiting for laughter. To hear it, feel it—be a part of it. I remembered that I owed that to others also.

*****

Tess
October 7, 2016

Life's greatest joys are my children…and sometimes their inability to stay that way!

Tess is with Nan at Applebee's.
October 7, 2016
Lubbock, Texas

Date night with a Florida mermaid!
Yup…they're letting the crazy squirrel out of the cage to go out to dinner!

Nan is with Tess.
October 7, 2016 at 9:16 p.m.

My date for tonight is singing karaoke…into the silverware!
#I'mTheOnlyOne #MelissaEthridge

Tom
October 7, 2016 at 5:17 p.m.

If you're the only one...you win!

Sally
October 9, 2016 at 12:18 a.m.

Tess, I did the same thing at Zip's with a french fry to "Man in the Mirror."
I totally feel ya, sister! XOXO
Patricia to Tess
October 8, 2016

Oh, my beautiful friend who makes the world a better place simply by being a part of it! She can deal with stress and carry heavy burdens. She smiles when she feels like screaming, and she sings when she feels like crying. She cries when she's happy and laughs when she's afraid. Her love is unconditional.

Hey Cancer...
You Picked the
Wrong Broad!

Janet
October 8, 2016

I'm no fan of the term *broad*, but this is so fitting for someone who has so much strength. Kick cancer's butt, Tess!

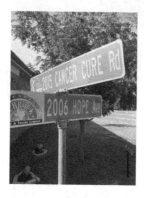

Tess
October 8, 2016

Nan's last day here, so we're going to attempt a walk on this cool autumn morning…

Just hanging out at the corner of cure and hope!

A beautiful day for a stroll through the Texas Tech Arboretum, maintained by the horticulture students. Weekends are my treatment breaks, so took advantage before rain scheduled to roll in.

Nan
October 9, 2016 at 9:08 a.m.

I will forever remember and treasure this beautiful walk we took together, my beautiful Tess!

*****

I was pushing it. I was so scared that I insisted on walking every day. I was not getting the sleep that my body and my mind needed, but at this point, I was afraid to sit still. I was afraid that if I stopped, so would my world. You may think that a silly or unproduc-

THE GRAY RIBBON WARRIOR

tive thought, but it creeps in, nonetheless. Fortunately, my caretakers were relentless on giving me hope, courage, and love.

*****

Tess
October 8, 2016

For some of the strong and caring Eagles in my life, who already know and live this… When we're in an "above" position of looking downward on others, it's so we can lift them up, not look down on them! Life is wonderful when we're looking eye-to-eye!

Tess
October 10, 2016

Day 1 of week 2 down… Kayla's first attendance with me. They told her she could take a picture tomorrow if we wanted.

I replied that there's already plenty pictures of angels on the Internet!

(This being in reference to the white blanket covering and the white mesh mask that pins my head to the table. I'm not thinking too many folks will be buying me as an angel…even for Halloween! LOL)

Monday morning visit with Doc. He said to start expecting an increase in the side effects this week, especially memory issues and fatigue…but as far as I'm concerned, each day completed is a day closer to being cancer-free and back in charge of my life!

*****

If the plan is to be in charge of my life, I've got quite a way to go!

In reality, I discovered that none of us have everything under control. Not really. And if I'm being honest, who would want to?

The best we can do is to control ourselves, and if we do that, we're doing great!

*****

Tess
October 10, 2016

Tonight was one of the nights when all can feel so much bigger than we can handle.

Pizza party night (for the time being, I still have the supersized appetite brought on by the steroids)... After Kayla and I sat down in the dining room with our dinner, I noticed an older gentleman sitting by himself, so I invited him to join the talkative twosome.

Turns out Gene and his wife have been married many many years, and he feels a bit overwhelmed with this being the first major crisis he and Carol have faced. She can't leave the hospital due to the severity of her treatments (her cancer is in the leukemia family), so he's staying here at the lodge alone.

It was crushing to watch his face as he talked, so much love for his wife and feeling fear for her. Watching everything they've created together change overnight... I understood for the most part, but know there are *huge* differences in our stories.

Since he's new here, I tried to make a few introductions and answer questions...but it surely doesn't feel like enough when someone looks so lost.

I am so grateful for the wonderful experiences and beautiful souls in my life. I truly believe a day will come that this will be behind me, and Tony and I will be living our adventures again with the people we love.

But if I could make one wish for all of us, it's that we recognize other people's fears, hardships, and journey as real and relevant for them, and that our hearts are willing to reach out and meet them on their path. Even if only for a moment!

Tess
October 10, 2016

Kirk
October 11, 2016

With so much of my Facebook page being taken up with negative causes, I want to thank my sister, Tess, for the encouraging words she writes every day in the face of her challenge (and her coming victory). And I thank all of her friends for rallying around her with encouragement and support and love. You are making a difference in her life.

Tess
October 11, 2016

I am not the face of cancer, and I will not let cancer be mine.

I don't have to pretend to be happy. There is so much good in life. But I will be honest... I do not feel brave; and in my opinion, the only reason I can even manage to show up for my treatments each day is the desire to continue watching that good in life. That good in you. And my children!

I am claustrophobic and have an anxiety disorder Having my head pinned down to a table every morning under a plastic mesh mask feels overwhelmingly suffocating. So I close my eyes, try to calm my breathing, and I don't move. The only way I can do this is to remember your words of encouragement.

I want to cry when I look in the mirror. My face is so swollen it's tight enough I could bounce a quarter off it (like they say with a soldier's bunk/bedding)...and I feel shame for my vanity.

The steroids have all but stripped me of my patience and temperament, for which my daughter often suffers the consequences; and yet she stands by my side, watching my every feeble move so I don't trip over my own feet (now that is brave...to watch your mother weaken daily!).

The brain surgery has messed with my memory and leaves me doubting myself often...and this is after the surgeon obviously did a phenomenal job!

I'm not brave. I don't think I have a choice.

But you do. And you choose to share your time. Wisdom. Confidence. Laughter. Strength. And you choose to *believe* in me and the power that watches over me.

I wish people could understand the power they hold within their hands, minds, and words, and use it for good instead of hurting each other.

All the political, personal, and religious battles we see on FB (and in life) could simply disappear because we are too focused on helping those truly in need.

Instead of talking about feeding the hungry, housing the homeless, curing diseases, and getting along...we just *do it.*

Now *that* is brave! Be *brave* today, my friend. All it takes to get started is showing up!

> Oh, Monday,
> You arrive, my faithful friend.
> You care little for the reputation,
> Deserved or not.
> Whether friends cheer,
> Or foes complain,
> You appear as promised
> Waiting for me to choose
> What I will do with you.
> I would do well
> To choose wisely...

Tess
October 12, 2016

Hump Day "jolt" done. Walked in to the radiation treatment room to Tom Petty coming through the speakers. Can't go wrong with that! I told the techs that today (in my imagination, under the mesh mask) I was going to the beach, and they were my cabana boys. I'm so blessed that they have a sense of humor! It's a sunny day here in Lubbock. I'll have to find a shady spot to sit back and enjoy it.

Escaped the loony bin for a bit. Thanks to Jerry and Nancy (friends from Lubbock Fraternal Order of Eagles). Kayla and I are enjoying fresh air, lunch, and laughs.

Tess
October 13, 2016

It's a beautiful, rainy day here in Lubbock…so I've finished getting chores done before my mom arrives tomorrow and am working on my writing.

Then this evening, we have volunteers from a local electric company coming in to barbecue up some dogs 'n' burgers…after which I hope to follow up with a guest violinist concert sponsored by Texas Tech University! Should make for the perfect rainy-day activities (not to mention a good night's sleep).

#IAcceptThatIHaveCancerButIWillNotLetItHaveMe

Tess
October 14, 2016

Yay! Friday has taken on a whole new meaning!

First *full* week of treatments completed; Mom arrives around noon, and we will head down the road so Mom can see our home in NM for the first time!

It's the perfect rainy day to spread a little of your particular brand of sunshine!

Have you ever tried to put makeup on a big ol' jack-o'-lantern? I personally have not. Until today. Yup, it's date night (with Willie Nelson, for sure!). And I wanted to look pretty for my guy…despite the fact that steroids have my face huge as a ripe fall pumpkin!

*****

85

One of the sweetest things Tony did for me was that he never made me feel bad about the way I looked. It seems to me that everyone understood that this was neither the place nor time for vanity. Everyone except me. But I was quickly learning that lesson. Before long, I truly could laugh at myself and thank my heavenly Father every day for standing by me through this!

*****

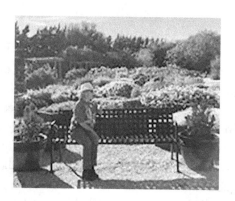

Tess
October 18, 2016

Mamasita enjoying a walk with me through the arboretum at TTU…a beautiful Texas day!

Tess
October 18, 2016

A long day ending with a perfect evening…

Volunteers made an amazing dinner of pulled pork, potato bar, and dessert choices included my favorite…cheesecake!

After dinner we hung out for *bingo* and then da da da daaaaa…3 new friends who brought so much joy and insight into my world! I cannot tell you ladies how much I appreciated you sitting with me and staying to visit! It's amazing how many blessings that can come out of difficult times!

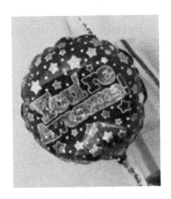

Tess
October 18, 2016

Way past bedtime… You know the insomnia is winning when you just sit and stare at the balloon follow you around the room like maybe it's trying to tell you something important! LOL

*****

I tried so hard to make light of my situation. Cancer is not light, but I was scared. So I poked humor at everything I did or said because it seemed so strange that I was doing and saying things that were not normal for me. My brain was creating its own stories to everyday things, and I was starting to lose sense of reality…or at least, what was real and what was made up by my brain. The brain didn't make up huge, fantastical stories; rather, they were everyday things that would make sense in the real world—but those things just didn't happen.

Although they seemed real enough to me, my partner knew that it wasn't, and it worried me all the more when he would correct me. He was quickly growing weary. I'm not sure I would have wanted to be in his shoes, but I was hurt and embarrassed; and at times, my response was mean. I would say things like, "I wish you could go through this, and then you'd understand!" In truth, I would never ever wish this horrible illness on anyone, much less someone I absolutely adore. He was correct, though. I wasn't myself anymore. I'm surprised he's still around.

Tess
October 19, 2016

I know there are people who can relate to just about every step I am going through, and there are those who are just trying to understand. This is why I share bits 'n' pieces of this journey.

To answer a few questions, I am on day...uhm...about 9 of radiation and chemo treatments, with about 25 days left of radiation. Not known yet as to how long chemo will continue after.

Everyone's reaction to treatment(s), thus story, is different.

That is something I didn't know going into this.

The side effects I am experiencing now are from the actual brain surgery and the medications, such as steroids. My radiation treatment is early in the game and differs a bit than other types of cancer, and as such, I'm not feeling the full-on attacks yet...and if I'm lucky, I may not.

I say all that because I know people are curious. Even all of us patients ask each other about our differences. It's okay to want to understand. But I don't feel strong or like a hero. I want to mention the people that I think are strong and act like heroes.

The strength it took my daughter, my friend Nan, and now my mother...to take time away from their lives so that I could fight for mine, makes me want to be a loving, caring, *strong* woman like them. It is not easy to watch someone you love suffer, but it surely takes strength to stand by their side while they do. (This is not intended to take away from those who would be here if you could. I understand responsibilities.)

And the volunteers who take time to come in, fix meals, and talk to patients who just want to have a chance at living...conversations like, "The world is still going around and *is* including you"... those are heroes because those people are saying, "You're worth my time!" And you know what? Every single one of us has the ability to be that kind of hero! Isn't that amazing? Just a bit of your time—

writing a note, prepping a meal, or having a conversation—and you become the hero you never knew was in you!

Today I met the only other brain cancer patient still around. He seemed the brave one to me. He is halfway through his treatments and has already suffered a stroke, leaving his left side crippled and blind in that eye. But he still smiled. And he still understood my fears and put on a brave face for me...a stranger. Very few words had to be exchanged to understand each other.

So you see, in my world, there has been no change of what I see as strong. Brave. Heroic.

Having said all that...

I do not spend any time in here watching the political election circus going on. Not just because the steroids have me as irritable as a pack donkey with a cactus stuck to his butt...but because I'm heartbroken over what we think matters and doesn't matter in this life.

I want to be so much more than I am. And everything happening in my life is leading me to different doors. Some I'm afraid to open because like any non-hero, I sometimes fear the unknown.

And yet everyday heroes keep "dropping" in to my life to remind me of a few basics:

1. No one's particular length of time here on earth is guaranteed, so make the most of every moment you are given, starting with making it the most for someone who needs you. Not one of those moments is ever a waste.
2. YOU ARE WORTH IT! But always remember...so are *they*.
3. Don't sweat the small stuff; that's what makes it the *big* stuff!

Hey! Thanks for hanging out with me for this long. Way to show your hero skills!

Tess
October 20, 2016

So excited to share!

Today I just completed (radiation) treatment 11...

That means I have made it almost a third of the way through! Woo-hoo!

I wish you could actually feel the smile I have on my face right now!

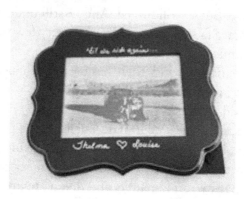

Making my room at the lodge feel like home...and my face smile!

Tess
October 20, 2016

"She is clothed with strength and dignity, and she laughs without fear of the future" (Prov. 31:25).

Yay, Friday is here! That means within the hour, Mom and I will be loading up the car and heading home for the weekend! I'm so excited to have a few days with my sweetheart and the usual "time off for good behavior!" It's a beautiful day for a weekend to start!

Tess
October 20, 2016

With a little bit of Ozzy and a lot o' bit of Downtown Tony Brown, we had a pleasant drive to Las Cruces and an enjoyable visit with Eagle friends.

Tonight is Tony and Stephanie's reception... Ready to cowgirl up!

Another beautiful New Mexico day!

*****

I was just happy to be with people who weren't sick or talking about dying. We were with friends celebrating life and love; and as exhausting as that was, it was needed. Tony kept pushing me. I think he was afraid I was going to give up, but I was tired; and as much as I wanted to see friends, I just wanted to sleep. But I didn't. I traveled, I mingled, and I even tried to dance once or twice. I needed to prove to myself that I could do it, and I needed to prove to him that I wasn't giving up so easily! But as always, I need to state that rest is so important to healing, and everything was taking its toll on me since I was not getting the rest I needed.

Tess
October 22, 2016

What a looooong day... I'm exhausted! At least I feel like tonight I'll sleep well!

It was a good day, and we had the joy of attending our friends' Tony V and Stephanie's wedding reception this evening. I had one dance with my sweetheart. It was all I could muster; but I didn't fall or puke on him, and it was perfect to see him smile. Recharged my heart and soul!

I think an hour in front of the firepit poolside to unwind and count my blessings will be just enough.

Now playing: "My Wish" by Rascal Flatts.

Tess
October 23, 2016

A very full and blessed weekend. Car is loaded and we're ready to make the four-hour drive home, where I will meet up with Mom and then head on back to Lubbock...where my home-away-from-home awaits.

Some days, a happy tired means everything! *But...* I look forward to the day I don't have to say goodbye to my sweetheart every Sunday afternoon.

Tess
October 24, 2016

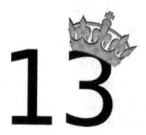

Woo-hoo! Treatment number 13 under the belt... Becoming an old pro at this!

My "happy mask" is getting tight. I'm pretty sure Kayla will be able to paint me a full-on jack-o-lantern face on it for Halloween!

(Biggest lesson in all this: finding joy and peace exactly where I'm at, never sitting around waiting for something better to come along!)

Today is about relaxing and enjoying the beautiful Texas weather!

Tess
October 28, 2016

Number 17!

That means today I may have hit the halfway mark for radiation! Woo-hoo!

My enthusiasm is not meant to downplay what people go through with treatments. It's awful, not fun!

But I celebrate that I am here in this world and even more so, that you are in my life!

We often talk about creating joy or happiness wherever we are, no matter the circumstances; but in the here and now, where I am at, I honestly feel it has been gifted to me. I did not have to work at creating it although work will surely follow.

Joy came to my door at a time I might choose to be bitter and angry, and I have been given new friends and exciting new projects to work on!

I can't wait to share the new projects with you, but it must wait just a bit longer although I hope you will find it to be worth the wait.

Have a safe and wonderful Friday night. Just do what you love!

Tess
October 28, 2016

We often talk about creating joy or happiness wherever we are, no matter the circumstances; but in the here and now, where I am at, I honestly feel it has been gifted to me. I did not have to work at creating it although work will surely follow.

Joy came to my door at a time I might choose to be bitter and angry, and I have been given new friends and exciting new projects to work on!

I can't wait to share the new projects with you, but it must wait just a bit longer although I hope you will find it to be worth the wait.

Have a safe and wonderful Friday night. Just do what you love!
XoX

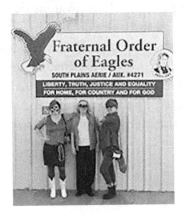

Tess
October 30, 2016

We escaped the Catt Cave for a few hours and got to have fun with our brothers and sisters in Lubbock! Zombie Cowgirl, Hope Jester, the Super Caregiver, and Rosie the Riveter!

*****

That night, at the Halloween party, I quietly talked to one of the ladies who had visited me at the hospital after my surgery. Her husband was in that day to have an outpatient procedure done. I vaguely remembered them visiting, but I told her I recalled walking the halls with them and that I had gotten so tired that I stopped at a nearby room where I saw an empty bed; then I crawled on to the bed, and I was embarrassed to wake up and see that everyone had just left me there. She looked at me with a bit of sadness in her eyes and said that, that never happened. She had stopped by to see me; but we didn't really get to converse much, and her husband wasn't with her.

It bothered me so much that I could somehow be creating a second reality. What if that became the norm for me? I had no idea how I was going to hide it, so I thought perhaps it was best to just not talk about things until others brought them up. Perhaps that's not the best approach since the doctors need to know everything that is going on, but what happens when you aren't sure what really happened or not? I guess my first thought would be to find someone you really trust, talk to them about "memories" that are coming up, and determine what is real and what isn't. Then you must let go of the false memories after you have talked to someone about them.

*****

Tess
November 2, 2016

Well, it has definitely been a Wednesday! So thankful to be headed toward the downhill!

Gather your chairs, kiddos. It's story time!

We just finished with dinner. The volunteers from a local church served fajitas, and we had a new couple (residents) join us at the table.

The wife has dementia. She kept grabbing Mom's food and offering to share with us. Then she stuck her fingers in Mom's fruit and started using the strawberries to illustrate her story.

I would say my momma's a saint; but seeing that she raised me, you already know the abundance of patience this woman has.

Despite my OCD of surviving dinner, they are a sweet couple with lots of fun stories (originally from Oregon). It's been an *interesting* and long day. Now I'm taking my bed meds, watching Food Network's *Worst Cooks in America*, and hoping to get a good night's sleep. Something I've come to miss.

Almost as much as I miss you! Sweet dreams from Texas!

*****

Dementia is not a laughing matter, and we were careful not to laugh in front of them. But later, Mom had to let me laugh out the events of our evening; otherwise, I would start crying. She knew that I pretty much had to laugh at everything or shrink away in fear. Can you imagine how frustrating it must be to be hungry but have a total stranger sticking their fingers into your food? I had started to become pretty obsessive-compulsive throughout all of this, but I was unsure if it was just my brain's reaction or everyone telling me how careful and clean I had to be to avoid getting germs since my immunity would be compromised.

While the husband was horribly embarrassed at first, with my mother's loving nature, she assured him that there was nothing to be embarrassed of; then she quietly moved her fruit plate over in front of the wife so she could continue to play happily in the food. Soon the husband was involved in conversation with us and would just casually reach over to correct her now and then so as to not draw attention.

Another gift I'd been given throughout this journey came in the form of the many amazing people I have been blessed to meet. We tend to walk around passing judgment on anyone different from us, especially if they think differently; but in reality, it is these differences that bring such beauty to this life!

Tess
November 4, 2016

Good morning, world!

I want you to know that I tried to give in to self-pity last night. Fatigue, pain, confusion…

But *you* wouldn't let me.

I tried to look in the mirror and focus with anger on the unrecognizable face, but instead was able to see your kind and patient eyes. Your laughing and loving smile. *You* gave me a chance at a beautiful new day today, and I will do my best to honor that gift.

If you ever want to doubt the existence of angels, just look at the people around you. Family, friends, and even strangers. Then look in the mirror.

Even when you feel your most unlovable, your angels will get you through!

Thank you for giving me hope in this new day… Thank you for being my angels!

Tess
November 7, 2016

It's another beautiful autumn day in Texas! The sun is shining, and we're supposed to hit 71 this afternoon… Don't you know I'll be out on a little walk for that!

Mom and I went home to NM over the weekend. So nice to have a couple nights in my own bed and time with my honey and my daughter.

Tony, his son Jesse, and I went to see the movie *Doctor Strange*. It's fun and funny…a great date movie, as well as good family time. (Don't misquote me here; I've never been a big fan of bringing the little ones to adult movies.)

I finished up for today with treatments and doc appointments. I seem to be doing exceptionally well. Since I'm just starting to really see and feel the effects beyond steroids, Mom and I took the time to go hat shopping to keep my head warm (and sun-free) since my hair is thinning but not coming out in clumps yet; and I'm starting to make changes to my dietary needs that will sustain me but slow down this rapid weight gain. (I have not yet had the loss of appetite many get during radiation/chemo since I haven't really come off steroids yet.)

Okay, the good news… Da da da daaaa… I hear there's only *ten* days left of radiation treatments!

I will be glad to be done. My head hates me for what I'm doing to it, but I feel really good about my medical team. So hopeful and positive!

A huge thank-you to all of you who have sent cards, PMs, prayers, and love. It warms the heart; and on the frequent-flyer insomniac nights, I roll over and look at the windowsill full of cards and do not feel alone.

I hope your week is off to as great a start as mine!

Love and prayers for my many friends and family out there going through their own hard times. Keep the faith, find the humor, and always, always find something positive to focus on!

Tess to Sherry
November 7, 2016

Thank you for always being there for me.

They left out the part in the Mommy Manual where it says, "You're stuck with us for life, not just the first 18 years."

I can't imagine going through this without you, but more important... I can't imagine what I promised to God before coming to earth that made him choose you to be our mother.

Whatever it was...it was worth it, and I hope I do it justice. I love you!

Tess
November 8, 2016

When you're done voting in America's Funniest Bloopers...er, uhm, I mean, presidential race...

May I ask you to take a moment to follow the link shown on this paper and cast a vote for the American Cancer Society Hope Lodge?

This is where I have been staying throughout my care, and other patients have come here from all over Texas and New Mexico.

Thank you for your time and consideration! It means literally the world to the many people they have helped!

In the meantime, whomever you chose to vote for in the US presidential race, please feel free to send your candidate to my Mary Kay skin care page. I think we could all agree they can both use a little lightening up!

*****

I will interject right here again. I had decided that selling skin care online would be my best option to keep money coming in. I was feeling guilty that Tony was the only one working, so I was certain that I could do this at least. In truth, I had so many memory and clarity issues that I could not keep it up, but the lesson to learn from this is to try and stay busy in a *positive* way.

A positive mindset absolutely helps. If all your loved ones are trying to remain positive for you, but you carry around a grudge toward the world, they will want to give up. When you find your happiness from within, in the midst of all the craziness, pain, and seemingly unbearable waiting, you will see that their courage and strength derive from you; and they can remain a rock for you on the days when they're really needed. Look for a hobby, or get back in to an old one. Keeping your mind and hands busy is crucial!

*****

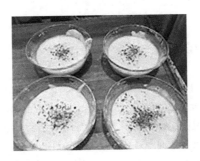

Tess
November 11, 2016

A wonderful homemade dinner by Master Chef Brown!

This lovely side dish was butternut squash soup made from scratch, veggies grown in our own garden! These days, I really *love* weekends!

A sneak peek into my next craft project...

We'll see how it turns out, but I'm excited to share the story with you as soon as it's done!

*****

I've always been a crafty person, not likely because I'm so good at it but more because I enjoy it and it's my "peaceful place." This is something you will need to do: find what makes you feel most peaceful, and plan on doing it. A lot.

*****

Tess
November 11, 2016

Because beauty may start in the eye of the beholder,
But it grows…in the hearts of those it is shared with.

Tess
November 15, 2016

Our week started off a little slow. One of the radiation machines was down, so I got delayed a treatment. But as of today, I am hopefully down to only four left…which means after a few follow-up appointments next week, Tony should be bringing Kayla and I home for good next Wednesday! (Chemo pill will continue from home; but I'll finally also be able to come off the steroids soon, I hope!)

Yesterday they had to do a biopsy on the tip of my nose, so we will be doing a multiple-step surgery soon to remove that skin cancer.

Their repeated apologies for having to do this on my nose was a fairly clear indication that they are not expecting me to be particularly pleased with the "cosmetic" outcome. But if even a handful of my friends use my experience to follow through and get yourself checked (from skin to boobs to prostate), it will totally make it worth the imperfection my nose will become!

Some days are better than others, but every day that we remember the "power of positivity" is a great day!

My hope is that soon I will be done with this forever and, more importantly, that we hit a time no one has to battle cancer!

Thank you for not leaving me to take this journey alone. It means more than you'll ever know!

*****

I had to come back to this particular post often. The doctor did an amazing job, but I didn't like the look of my nose afterward. I had to remind myself that my vanity was not worth my life; and in truth, he had done an excellent job. I had seen others' results, and it was what kept me holding off from getting it done when I should have earlier.

*****

Our week started off a little slow…one of the rad machines was down so I got delayed a treatment…but as of today, I am down to only four left…which means after a few follow-up appointments next week, Tony should be bringing Kayla and I home for good next Wednesday!!! (Chemo pill will continue from home but I'll finally also be able to come off the steroids)

Yesterday they had to do a biopsy on my nose, so we will be doing a multiple-step surgery soon to remove that skin cancer. Their repeated apologies for having to do this on my nose was a fairly clear indication that they are not expecting me to be particularly pleased with the outcome…but if even a handful of my friends use my experience to follow through and get yourself checked (from skin to boobs to prostate), it will totally make it worth the little imperfection my nose will become!

Some days are better than others…but every day that we remember the "power of positivity"…is a great day!!!

My hope is that soon I will be done with this forever, and more importantly, that we hit a time no one has to battle Cancer!

Thank you for not leaving me to take this journey alone… It means more than you'll ever know!

Tess
November 17, 2016

Today was Mom's last day with me. She flies home tomorrow and finally gets to see/enjoy the progress on her forever/retirement home with my brother and his wife on the other side of Washington State.

Tony drove Kayla out to take Mom's place with me for my last week at the lodge. I have only two more scheduled radiation treatments then follow-up labs and appointments. And if all goes well, Tony will be bringing Kayla and I home for the last time on Thanksgiving morning. How awesome is that?

I mentioned that they "biopsied" my nose, and it did come back positive for skin cancer; and they have scheduled me mid-December for a day-long surgery in which they plan to remove parts of my nose section by section, each time running it through the lab. And if the section doesn't come back free of cancer, they go back and remove another section...until they come back with a clear slice.

Yesterday, the radiation team encouraged me to talk to my different doctors and consider the option of radiation instead of surgery. I will make my decision some time next week, hopefully based on which option gives me a better chance of *not* being a repeat customer. As awesome as the medical team at UMC/SW Cancer Center is... I'd just as soon see them at a fundraiser or church event than looking up at them through a plastic mesh mask, pinning me to a cold iron slab. I do not envy them their jobs. It takes a strong person to keep a positive bedside manner...and a winning attitude to humor my craziness!

In the meantime, tonight is for relaxing and focusing on all the joy and adventures that lay ahead! And what better way to do it than music? Tonight it is a CD put out by our lovely Nan Riddle (YouTube). Makes my heart happy!

Take time every day to visit what makes you happy. Then share it with all the love you have in your heart!

*****

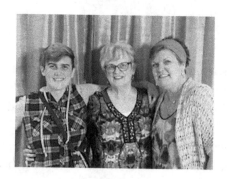

When it came time for Mom to leave, I was sad but also thankful that I had my daughter to stay with me at the Hope Lodge. We took a picture before Mom left, something I was avoiding, along with all the weight gain; but we wanted to document the memory. The truth is no one really ever made me feel bad about my weight gain. I should have given my friends and family much more credit. Anytime I saw any of them, they just helped me up and down cars, chairs, stairs, etc., without saying a negative word.

Tess
November 20, 2016

The Catt in the Hat

Honestly, I've lost track of how long I have been here at the lodge (time and I are sort of strangers these days)… But after all this time, I've just found out that for those who didn't know my name, I'm referred to as the girl in the hat. Many around here do wear hats, but why I stick out to the other patients is because I still have hair and yet wear hats.

Around here, patients learn to get comfortable asking each other questions that non-patients might feel uncomfortable asking. We learn that all cancers and all patients are not the same. Treatments are not the same, and thus, side effects are not the same. Who knew?

So back to my hats. The wind blows here most all the time, and whether I'm heading out with damp hair for my early-morning treatments, or the afternoon sun is shining…due to the fact that my radiation treatments are directly through my scalp, my head is tender; and I simply try to keep it from direct contact with Mother Nature.

Since my chemo comes in pill form, the odds were I wouldn't lose all my hair like many others. It is thinning; and due to the radiation, my hair isn't currently growing on the surgical site. And like many others having radiation, the site is left feeling "raw and sunburned" and, of course, the uncomfortable swelling. Thus… I hide "the vulnerable" behind my hats.

It's really not a big deal; but in the insomnia hours, a girl (with or without hats) has a lot of time on her hands to think.

We all at some point try to hide our vulnerabilities because we see them as weaknesses.

This got me thinking about my life and the changes I want to make if the good Lord decides y'all have to put up with me for years to come.

And while it's not likely I'll uncover my head and leave it to the discomforts of Mother Nature just yet... I have to admit I've grown weary of feeling the need to apologize to others for my "weaknesses."

In truth, we learn that there are just some folks out there that thrive on finding people's weaknesses and exposing them.

But...what if I stopped seeing these things as my weaknesses, and I focused on making them a strength?

*****

This particular day's post was brought on by a fellow patient staying at the Hope Lodge. I do not know what her type of cancer was, but she also wore hats and seldom smiled. I honestly can't blame her for that as there is so much that's bad in cancer and the treatments; but on this particular day, she was really snapping at everyone, mostly at her daughter.

Out of the blue, she turned to me and ripped the hat off her head, exposing her balding scalp. She had chosen not to cut her hair or shave her head, so she had a few straggly clumps of long hairs left. She pointed at her own head and said something to me to the effect of "You don't belong here! You wear hats every day and yet still have so much of your hair!" She was very angry, and I reminded myself that it wasn't particularly directed at me. But I admit that my emotions were all over the place by this point, and I had to work very hard not to cry in front of everyone in the dining area.

I wasn't sure what to say. She had never seen me before this stay; so she did not realize that I was losing my hair (just not all over my head) and that I had already put on over twenty-five pounds from the steroids. It hurt. I didn't want to be the outcast of the group, but I was honestly so grateful that I was not doing as bad as Doctors were expecting. In fact, they seemed quite pleased with themselves over my results. Somehow, to me, this seemed to feel unfair to some other patients.

I'm not sure how many people realize the effects of the little things they say and do, especially when you feel like you are all alone in the world though surrounded by many. After that last interaction, I went to my room, stepped into the shower and cried alone for a short bit. Then I cleaned myself up and crawled under a warm blanket to read. The last thing I wanted was to feel sorry for myself.

*****

Tess
November 20, 2016

My daily strength: "Prayer of Thanks. Father, help me to love and appreciate the person *you* created me to be. I thank you that I don't have to compare myself to others in order to be accepted. *You* created me with a unique and wonderful purpose. I'm thankful that to *you* I am special and beyond compare."
~ Joyce Meyer, *The Power of Being Thankful: 365 Devotions for Discovering the Strength of Gratitude*

*****

Here, I would like to give a big thank-you to Facebook. It has opened up a whole new avenue of communication wherein people can cause damage…or build communities. Full of strength, love, and fellowship. It's always in the little things we say and do that make something good or bad.

*****

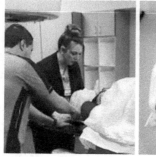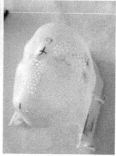

Tess
November 21, 2016

Eeeeek!
Done, done, diddly done!
Radiation treatments to the brain are done!
They marched me out of the treatment room to the song "Celebrate" and a standing ovation with bubbles and "flying" streamers. I didn't want to cry like a baby, but the tears went silently down my cheeks... I'm overwhelmed with joy!
So my graduation present was the mask of torture. Please feel free to offer ideas on what to do with it! LoL

*****

As of the date of this "in-between writing," the mask of torture currently sits on a shelf in the garage, waiting for me to decide what to do with it. I've thought about making it a jewelry holder, but part of me wants to toss it. It's not just a reminder of what has happened (which is nothing short of miraculous); but it is also a reminder that it could happen again on any day. In fact, most people are curious and want to ask about my journey; but even more so, they want to share about their family member's experience dealing with cancer... and the outcome.
While staying in the Hope Lodge, I waited to hear a story of someone having brain cancer who did well or even survived for more

than a couple years. It breaks my heart every time someone wants to share their story. I know they need to, so I listen and love; but in truth, it scares me. I have unfinished business in life…but then again, don't we all?

Tess
November 21, 2016

Guess where I am? Do you know?
Go ahead!
Just sitting on the corner of *joy* and *chill!*
I'm home and happy, happy, happy!
Home-cooked meal under way by that handsome man!

Tess
November 23, 2016

Thank you for your kindness, patience, and love. Sometimes we forget just how much we can do for others just by giving a bit of ourselves and our time. You literally change the world, even if only for one person at a time.

Many have asked where it goes from here for me.

For now, I rest and rebuild.

My labs and MRI are scheduled in early December, at which time we will see if everything is gone.

There are no guarantees in life except one: God will be there through it all, if you ask him to.

No promises that it will be easy, but I truly believe he gives us each other to get through the tough times and celebrate *all* times!

Why we fight that, I'll never really know. I mean, a world full of life, creativity, and ability to love…and we nitpick the joy out of living.

Not today.

Today I celebrate whatever time I have left on this earth. Today I will be grateful for what my friends and "enemies" alike have taught me (and believe me, if you fall in to the enemy category, you have the ability to pull out of it just as you chose to go in it).

Today I will put my clothes and belongings away into my own drawers and closet and be thankful I have a home.

But mostly, I will be thankful for you. What you bring to my life and this world!

It's okay. I know I'm a sappy kind of girl. I have bad days like everyone; but I've learned to cry it out in private, if I need to at all… then just be happy. I'm not telling you what to do. I'm just sort of sharing life through my perspective.

In my world (the activities that I choose to do and, in truth, the world at large), there will always be someone to tell you what you're doing wrong, what is wrong with you…

But I want to tell you it will be okay. Just be you. You were designed with purpose, so why fight it?

Despite what some say, you're not always doing it wrong. You're doing it you. If you do anything out of *love*, it's surely going to do someone some good but especially you. And it's okay to love *you*. It makes it easier to love others!

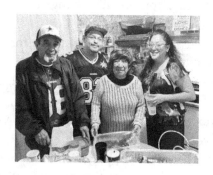

Tess
November 24, 2016

Happy Thanksgiving!
Fredrica, from the bottom of our hearts… Thank you.

I'm so sorry I'm just such a deadhead right now. I want so much to get back to living a normal life, and I push it. But everyone concurs...outstanding meal and even "outstanding-er" people!

I'm so looking forward to getting healthy enough I can start joining the workouts at your club, and it will be great if we can pull together that girls' craft night!

Love you to pieces!

Tess
November 24, 2016

Bedtime...

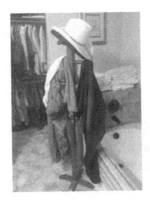

A quick funny before I collapse for the night...

This coat tree has been freaking me out since I got home from Lubbock.

Between steroids and radiation to the brain, I've had side effects to my vision.

My peripheral is bad, and up-close vision is extremely blurry. (Still a lot of swelling in the noggin'.)

But we got home from a wonderful Day of Thanks celebration with the Flores family, and I have walked by this thing at least a dozen times again.

My last stop in to the closet, I spin around quickly, not really paying attention.

Holy Moses, I must have jumped three feet in the air! Once again, my brain was turning it in to a living person. Thankfully this Catt landed on her feet!

Seriously, I literally said, "Oh, excuse me!"

*Sigh… I really have to laugh at myself because I'm pretty sure you'd be laughing if you'd seen me!

Sweet dreams, my friends. Be sure to carry all of the joys of today in to the new day tomorrow! Let go of the sadness of yesterdays!

Tess
November 25, 2016

Yum!
Thanksgiving leftovers! Breakfast of champions!

Tess to Tony
November 27, 2016

"Sleeping next to someone you love makes you fall asleep faster, reduces depression, and helps you live longer."

I'm so happy to be home. If this is true, I will always seek to be by your side!

Tess
November 29, 2016

Kick-starting a new week!

We are fooling ourselves if we think we are living in a time when "dirty politics" have become the norm. It's been around as long as Adam and Eve.

We are still seeing it at the highest level and are watching it trickle down into our everyday lives. Our relationships, our jobs, our streets, and our organizations.

We "accept" it because we convince ourselves there isn't anything we can do about it.

It seems to me a miracle we have survived this long as we seem hell-bent on destroying ourselves.

Call me Captain Obvious; but it also seems to me that despite our selfishness, greed, and sometimes dishonorable intentions…that there is a reason we are still here regardless of all our attempts to do ourselves in. A reason much larger than any of us individually but as a collective, gives us cause to celebrate.

So I offer you this challenge: please take a moment to reflect on a purpose (reason) you feel that *you* as an individual are here for and what you can do to fill that purpose.

Then…celebrate that purpose by *doing* whatever you feel it takes to fulfill that purpose.

This assignment, should you choose to accept it, will not expire, explode, or self-destruct in thirty seconds… But if you have chosen a positive and productive way to meet *and fly* with your "purpose," the odds are in your favor that you will see miracles of positive proportions!

♪ Don't believe me? Just watch!
Welcome to Monday, my friends! ♪

Tess to Sherry
November 29, 2016

Of all the "memories" to get stuck in my head… I'm "hearing" the sound of that elevator's "bells" (from the Hope Lodge)! LOL.

*****

Memories. We often forget how important they are until we don't have access to them anymore. This was quickly becoming an even scarier time for me than the brain surgery itself. To the medical team, I was pretty much a walking miracle. To me, I felt lost and alone.

By this point, I was full into feeling the cancer and treatment side effects. Oftentimes, I couldn't even be sure that the memories were real or if my "new brain" was making them up. I could remem-

THERESA CATT

ber things from before the surgery and the treatments if someone reminded me, but what I was starting to find is I had difficulty with the short-term memory. And edema stinks!

I also did not like looking in the mirror, and obviously this wasn't going to correct itself, much less overnight. There were times I could overhear my partner explaining my appearance to others. I was not in control of my emotions, so that hurt. I felt embarrassed and sad that Tony was stuck explaining. Sometimes I could see the hurt in his eyes. Couldn't people just accept me no matter how large or small I was? I wanted to scream that the physical changes weren't permanent, but the truth was that I didn't know.

In reality, people did accept (if not, feel bad for me); and the love was pouring in. But you can't always tell at the moment if your brain is playing with you. I didn't want pity; I wanted acceptance—not of the cancer but of me as a human being and where I was in this whole journey. This will always be a need in most of our lives. Cancer or not.

Tess
December 1, 2016

I blinked...and 2016 is almost gone!

Just a quick note to thank you all for joining me on my last "adventure" of the year. It is, of course, attempting to ride along with me into the new year, but I have plans of my own!

I have finished off most meds and treatments for now, and the side effects are slowly starting to taper. I did go in to the doc yesterday in quite a bit of pain and have been put on antibiotics for an infection.

Honestly, I'm tired. But even bigger than that, I'm grateful you were here, cheering me on. It is people like you that are the true heroes.

Because you help the weary cross the finish line.

You give harmony when the music stops playing.

And you bring laugher and smiles when the body wants to quit.

Never forget your value in this world, and let's do everything we can to make 2017 a year of positive change and growth!

*****

I had not realized that this was not the end. I heard that I was going to have up to years of ongoing issues from the treatments, but I am praying that the cancer never returns. As much as I am trying to exercise and eat healthy, the hardest thing for me to stay away from is sugar. As I understand, sugar is what feeds cancer cells. It thrives on it. I've been trying to stay on top of taking my daily "shot" of apple cider vinegar. I also received a healthy-recipe book from my friend...

*****

Tess to Debi
December 1, 2016

I'm so excited to dig in and eat/live well!
(And shed this other woman who's trying to live in my skin with me! LOL)
Love you! Thank you!

Tess
December 3, 2016

I just want to cross the finish line and be done with this life-triathlon.
Having said that, I told you that my MRI was scheduled for Monday (12/5), at which time we would know the results of all the treatments.
However, there was a death in that medical department, so they will shut down Monday for the funeral and rescheduled me to Monday 12/12. (Understandable.)
Until then...life as normal as my body will allow.

Although I have decided that after the tests, I will never be normal since I have not been that since, like, the third grade. So back to being stranger-than-life Tess…with a few changes.

#LetDateNightCommence #RemindingMyselfEveryDayThat ThisTooShallPass

Tess
December 3, 2016

After a couple of nasty days, today I managed to get a few things done. But for tonight, I'm asking Mr. Speedy Gonzales to sit down and snuggle in front of a movie. Wait… Are we the only ones who don't have Christmas decor up yet?

*****

It was becoming apparent that my partner was staying as busy as possible, mostly away from me. I took this very personally—that at a time when I needed to feel loved, he was pulling away. In reality, he was just keeping busy himself. We were taking one hit after another, and he was doing his best to keep his head above the waters of despair.

*****

Tess
December 09, 2016

As mentioned, my MRI is rescheduled for the 12th, and we'll find out if all the cancer is gone from the brain. The 14th, I am scheduled for surgery for the cancer on my nose.

And on the 21st, I start a new round of chemo. It's still pill form, 3 times the previous dose; but I only take it one week a month (so have a three-week break between each time). This is for six months, I believe. I've been told it will have the same "kick" as if I were receiving it intravenously, so it should do the trick.

I get to stay home this time during the chemo, so my husband now becomes Nurse Tony.

But...the last few days have been good! Some relief from pain and nausea, seeing my daughter get the help she needs, a bit of Christmas shopping, *and* I got lunch at Five Guys the day before and a dinner date with the number one guy last night. (I can tell already it's going to be a slow-go to get him on board with my weight-loss plans! LOL!) I suppose if I just stick to his pickled beets, I may be successful.

The really cool part is that we pick Teresa up at the airport today! Yup, it's going to be a *Thelma & Louise* weekend! (No guns or cliffs involved, of course...and Louise is a bit of a gimp this weekend! Haha!)

HAPPY FRIDAY, LUVS!

Tess
December 12, 2016

Well, boo on the medical team!

I was originally scheduled for the 5th to get my MRI (see if all the cancer in the brain is gone); then they rescheduled me to the 12th (I even have the voicemail from the 9th reminding me of my appointment). I drove to Lubbock...and they said, "You don't have an appointment. We rescheduled you to January 19."

Soooo sad! I really would like all of this to be over, and I'm not thrilled about waiting another month.

The worst part is that we took Teresa to the airport today... and had I known they had rescheduled me, I could have called Rob and told him, "I'm so sorry, but I'm kidnapping your wife. You must come here and spend some time with us too in order to get her back!"

I'm telling ya, this was not a win-win day! Bright side: nice weather, and I'm wrapping the grandkids' Christmas presents!

Tess
December 14, 2016

What a beautiful view for our drive early this morning to Lubbock! Father in heaven, give me courage.

I realize that some people get a tad annoyed when I talk about skin cancer and the importance of getting checked. But it's a reality that anyone could have to face, so I'm just asking you to at least teach your kids to use sunscreen; and most importantly, don't use the tanning beds. It *is* possible to tan with sunscreen, but even one sunburn can cause permanent damage. See a dermatologist; they can give you information!

I have pictures from the MOHS surgery because Tony was able to stay in the room during the procedure—a great comfort—and he was able to help get all the instructions. (And thank you to our sweet friend Fredrica for offering to help me. Literally, up until this morning I didn't want to go!)

But my reasoning here is that I don't want to see anyone suffer needlessly or "for the sake of beauty" when you are already beautiful!

I'm not asking for pity. I'm doing everything I can to get healthy again, and I am grateful for the amazing support that has been shown to me. I am just asking you to be careful and be healthy! Stick around awhile, and do great things!

Keep your heart beautiful, and you will be seen as beautiful all the way around!

Tess
December 15, 2016

Some days, ya just gotta laugh it out and be thankful.
For example…
Whenever I start missing the home I owned,
the water softener goes, the dishwasher blows,
the kitchen floods, and I ruin my duds.
The Christmas lights don't work,
The mailman is late (I mean he, not she)
I miss my kids… And the "free shipping" wasn't free!

And then...
A neighbor stops by with Christmas snacks,
A friend I miss gives a pat on my back.
I hear my sweetheart's calming voice,
and remember my choice.
Rejoice, rejoice!
I catch a glimpse in the mirror
It's not as bad as could I fear...
I could be a snail, always carry my home,
Leaving trails of...oh, good grief...wherever I roam.
I could be washing dishes by campfire (oh, wait... I like that!)
But I could be a Grubb instead of a Catt!
It's all-in perspective,
I see that quite clear...
I could be you (reading this horrible little poem)
Instead of bending your ear!
Happy Thursday, Luvs!

Tess
December 17, 2016

Don't be sad if you're having snowy/freezing weather. Just remember...
You are the sunshine on a dreary day!

*****

I was starting to feel better. Or at least, I thought I was. I even believed that I was going to get to bypass all the horrible side effects that others were (or had been) dealing with. I suppose that if I were honest, I would not have wanted to know all of this ahead of time; but the truth is a little knowledge beforehand allows a cancer patient to feel less of a victim and more of a warrior! In reality, it might take time and could still get worse from here.

Tess
December 19, 2016

We are seeing many (FB) reposts that I think are wonderful. It *is* the time of year we usually take the extra time to think of, pray for, and help out people in need.

It seems odd then that the rest of the year, we watch people bullying, cheating, and intentionally harming others.

"Sticks 'n' stones" may be a pleasant little ditty we teach our children to toughen up; but the truth is, we wouldn't use our words as weapons if it didn't work.

This 2016 seemed like an exceptionally harsh year. (the US presidential campaign being a very real and sad example.)

While "Peace on Earth" is a pleasant greeting we send each Christmas season, it seems to me that if we want it to be a reality, it starts in our homes. Our workplaces and schools. Our organizations.

In our own hearts.

Tess
December 21, 2016

For those who are friends with Kayla/Kiki and wondered if she disappeared…

She is in the hospital but is doing well.

Having had her thyroid removed and a hysterectomy all within this last year has taken its toll.

They have pulled her off most meds to determine what she needs or does not and had to reduce her thyroid med dosage since she had gone the other way.

If you truly know her, you know that she's a loving soul; but the last few months have brought depression and chaos for her, and she was just finally ready to give up the fight.

We got to see her Monday night and talk on the phone last night; and she's starting to sound more like her spirited old self, but with a bit more understanding of what she'll need to do for herself to have the life she wants.

Today I'm headed to Lubbock to get stitches out of my face. Tonight I'll be back to see Kayla and see if she recognizes her own Momma! LOL

She doesn't have Internet access right now as far as I know, but feel free to leave her a note here or send a PM. She'll see them soon when she gets home.

*****

My cancer, along with all of its side effects, wasn't just taking its toll on me; but it was affecting those whom I love, who were there to see it and had to deal with it. I was exhausted trying to take care of myself and help my daughter, but it gave me something to focus on since I had lost just about all ability to focus at this point.

You hear about the harshness of the treatments, but it all gets brushed aside when you hear those words, "You have cancer." I only knew that I was scared and wanted to live and would do anything the doctors told me to ensure that I could stay around for my loved ones. Just not the currently brain freak that I felt like I was.

I felt horrible. I had already lost most of my hair in the area I called the halo, which is where the radiation entered and exited the skull. I was heavier than I had been in my entire life and was missing most of one eyebrow and half the other, and most of my eyelashes were dropping. Whatever hair that was left anywhere was thinning. On the bright side, I didn't need to shave as often. Yes, all my friends also thought, *TMI*; but the point here is to share just one person's story.

*****

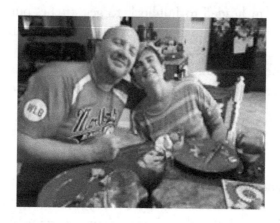

Tess—with Sherry and 3 others.
December 25, 2016

My Christmas, dinner dates!

Tony made both turkey and ham for the three of us, with oyster stuffing… Yummy!

Kayla and I made banana/cranberry bread from scratch. We'll see if we can even come close to Mr. B's cooking. Now…to find me a mental hammock on a warm beach!

Merry Christmas, Luvs!

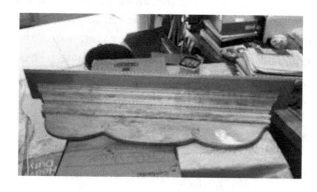

Tess to Sherry
December 25, 2016

Belated Merry Christmas and happy retirement!

Just finished putting first coat of polyurethane on to protect it.

Tony did all the construction and trimming; Kayla carved the "swirls"; and I do the finish, as usual.

When it's dry, we'll add the beautiful dragonfly hooks...and you have your garden-themed shelf!

We should have it in shipping on Wednesday.

Apologies for being late, but please know how much we love you! Tony, Tess, and Kayla.

*****

Tony and Kayla encouraged me to take it easy but to keep doing the little projects I loved so much, if I felt up to it.

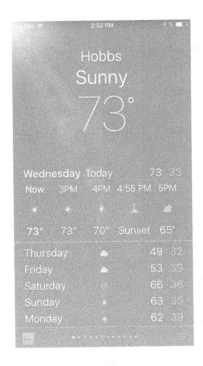

Tess with Kayla
December 28, 2016

I was in a hurry this morning but not feeling well; so as I was rushing out the door, I grabbed a jacket and scarf and threw them on. (Right now, I wear a hat nearly every day because direct cold or heat irritate the parts of my scalp that are bare or had surgery.)

I got in the truck and figured it was so warm because the heater was on from yesterday.

Everyone stared as I walked in the phone shop. I'd like to say it was my charming smile...but the attached photo will explain better ;)

Needless to say, they were really laughing when I started stripping off all the layers but insisted on leaving the hat on!

Home now and trying to enjoy the nice weather while I can. Tomorrow we're heading toward cooler parts!

Tess
January 01, 2017

Happy 2017!

No matter what this year brings, what we make of it is what we have to live with!

I got to spend an icy-cold weekend with some of Nebraska's finest, and I danced into 2017 with my honey! (Okay, it was only two dances, but it was more than I thought I'd be able to do!)

Tess to Frederica
January 01, 2017

Okay, it slowed down a bit today. We fly home tomorrow, and I need to see you about joining the fitness class. For some reason, a lot of my side effects have hit "late"; and although I was already gaining weight, I am having trouble with really sore muscles and joints and stability (literally, people are having to help me stand/sit/walk). I'm hoping if I get going, I can get some strength back and start *living* again! XOX

Tess
January 02, 2017

Over the last few weeks, the side effects of the treatments/medications have really started kicking in. The last few days, emotions really took a hit. I have had an overwhelming feeling of sadness/loneliness (which is beyond wrong because I have got to spend that time with some really awesome family, which truly helped me from losing it altogether).

So the only thing I could think of was my sorrow over losing 2016.

Not!

Believe me, I am grateful for every day that I am given… although I definitely see no reason to look back. I have learned a lot of lessons over the last few months (like realizing that I am either truly vain or fear judgment). But I have been overwhelmed with blessings and love; and if there is one thing I can do in 2017, that would be to spread those blessings and love!

The best thing I plan to carry over in to this year are the friendships and family!

*****

By now, I was understanding what other cancer survivors were talking about, and my main worry was that I was never going to be the same. Would I be able to dance again? Would I be the strong multitasker and organizer I was before? Would I even be able to follow the simplest of instructions? (As I am writing this part more than a year later, I must say that I still have the aches and pains of neuropathy and tinnitus, as well as some clarity and memory issues.)

Here and now, I have stopped worrying so much about what will happen because in reality, it's in God's hands. I do not like pain, and I do not like having to be dependent. I learned at the early age of five years old to not like needles. But still…it could have been far worse. I have come to believe that I *am* the walking miracle that people say I am. That does not make me a superhero; but it just means that as much as I feel some days like I have really suffered, it's not even comparable to some others.

*****

Via Messenger

Tess,

One last dose of chemo, huh? How brave of you to go through such of a journey! Like I have said, you have been in my thoughts and prayers, and I have hoped all was well. I am very proud of you for going through all of this. I know you haven't been alone, but I am sure you have felt that way at times. Your determination has pulled you through, and pretty soon the roses you once smelled will smell even sweeter. God is good, and God is good all the time.

Sometimes we don't understand what life brings to us, or we feel its unfair; but for each of us, it's how we pull through, handle, tackle, and learn from it that will take us down a new path—a better path. That path may have humps and bumps too; but we know how to handle them, and the people we meet along the way help guide us. Life's beautifully constructed and always goes on... We are the road signs that block our past.

You are almost done and like you said, done forever. I will help pray for you that it is. You have endured enough. Your gold heart and jovial personality need to spread and shine. Misti.

*****

This little note is included because I feel it's important to share the power of God's love. This woman and I were not necessarily friends although we did have a couple small things in common. I decided that it was best not to share the first communications between she and I because it was very personal. She was the woman whom my children's father first became involved with, thus helping us on to the divorce that was needed.

After I had moved down South, I had received the first note from her in her attempt to make amends and for both of us to move on with our lives. She did not know that through all the pains and frustration of my illness and treatments, God had taught me a deeper love—a truer understanding of each of our need to forgive and be forgiven. I had already forgiven her for my sake, and now it was time to let her know. Life has since moved on.

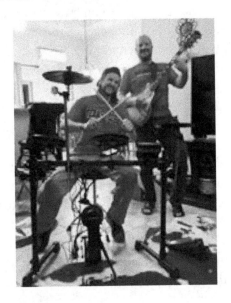

Tess
January 07, 2017

A new band in town…the Texas Browns.
What's the title of their new chart-topping country-rock song?

*****

I haven't mentioned Jesse for a bit here. He had surgery, wherein they removed one-third of his right lung (the lower lobe). The doctors here in town decided, however, that Jesse did not need follow-up radiation or chemotherapy. He came along quite quickly in his recovery and, in no time, was taking college classes and working. This young man meant business! However, cancer had its own designs.

Jesse and I both knew that we had to move forward. It was difficult for some people to understand that he and I both had a rough journey ahead of us, but we were on different paths. As I had said before, every person's story is different because every cancer is different. We handle the treatments individually while some folks have the same basic side effects. Also, where you have cancer in your body can cause different reactions. His lung cancer turned out to be from the sarcoma, which had been hidden away in his body for ten years then made a vicious return at the ripe old age of nineteen. But that is not my story to tell.

My cancer, being in the brain, affected many areas because your brain runs everything. In my early fifties, I was looking to a brave young man, who showed confidence and so little fear (if any) to people on the outside of his world, no matter how he felt on the inside. That does not mean, however, that neither of us never felt angry or, at some points throughout, abandoned. But to put it into perspective, this was (and is) our lives. While others continued living theirs, we felt left behind though no one ever really left us.

I will say that Jesse overcame cancer *twice*; and as I write, he is now on his third. He is a true warrior on the battlefield of this thing we call life.

Tess with Tony
January 09, 2017

It was a nice day for a walk around the pond!

The surface was frozen. (You can see where the kids threw big rocks at the water, and they're "magically" floating.)

When I arrived, a gaggle of geese met me at the car. Luckily, I had a tiny bit of food. I threw it and scurried away like the gimpy kitty I am right now. They were waiting for me when I arrived back at my car (1/2 mile).

I jumped in the car fast as I could, being careful not to catch any of them in the door. As soon as I shut it, they started "pecking" at the wheels.

Don't tell Tony, but I'm pretty sure his evil parrot Bilbo sent them after me! LOL

Tony stayed behind to work on another project while he has the awesome weather.

*****

The best thing I could do for myself was get out of the house each day, even if only for a walk around the block. I most enjoyed being out in nature, and this "lake" in the middle of the park just a few miles from the house was perfect. Another important thing is finding a happy place away from the home. I had not yet realized what a miracle this had all been. I was actually walking around the lake by myself, and it felt amazing!

In reality, I should not have been out there on my own at all. Yes, there were a few others at the park, but I didn't really have a good mental grasp on what my body was going through or would still be going through for months—and maybe even years—to come. I only knew that I was so happy to be enjoying God's beautiful work. Even if I could no longer run my laps around the lake or even keep a slow and steady walking pace, I was still walking when many in the medical field had warned that I might not be able to. At least not as soon as I had been able to.

*****

Tess to Shay
January 08, 2017

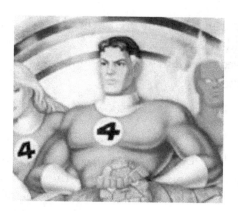

Sheesh! Hope my hair turns out as cute as yours as (if) mine grows back!

I'm mainly losing (lost) the hair directly where the radiation went in my head…and what hasn't fallen out yet in that area is not all gray/white but sort of "void" of color. Of course, that's at the sides around the ears, so I look like that cartoon character in *Fantastic Four*.

I'd laugh at myself if I wasn't me! Nope. I'm still laughing.

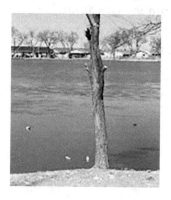

It was a nice day for a walk around the pond! The surface was frozen. (You can see where the kids threw big rocks at the water, and they're "magically" floating.)

When I arrived, a gaggle of geese met me at the car. Luckily, I had a tiny bit of food. I threw it and scurried away like the gimpy kitty I am right now. They were waiting for me when I arrived back at my car (1/2 mile).

I jumped in the car fast as I could, being careful not to catch any of them in the door.

As soon as I shut it, they started "pecking" at the wheels.

Don't tell Tony, but I'm pretty sure his evil parrot Bilbo sent them after me!

Tony stayed behind to work on another project while he has the awesome weather—with Tony Brown.

Tess with Kayla
January 10, 2017

Some men aren't meant to be dads, but every little girl is meant to be loved!

I am so grateful for Tony, stepping up to show you what matters in life. His willingness to dance, cook, and garden with you and call you family. And Tom, who willingly stepped in as godfather, giving you his friendship, listening ear, and time (coffee dates). And Geoff, who is sharing his world, heart, and friendship with you.

Not all men are great. None of them are perfect. But you deserve what each of these men have given of themselves. And you will always have me and your brother! I love you, Angel Face.

Tess
January 10, 2017

The clouds have moved in, but it's still supposed to make it to 70 today! I'm so grateful for the bit of warmth. The cold had been really hard on my body. (Thank goodness for all the warm hearts I have in my life!)

Speaking of which… I go back to Lubbock tomorrow for more labs and a follow-up with my oncologist. Then on Friday, I return for the elusive MRI, which should give me the results of the surgery and subsequent treatments. (Is the cancer gone?)

I laughed a bit about it being on Friday the 13th, but how were they to know…my favorite number/day! I have faith it's going to be my best Friday the 13th ever!

Regardless of the MRI results, the docs want me to continue chemotherapy for the next 6–12 months. I will make this choice when I come to it.

Tess
January 11, 2017

A beautiful day for a sort-of-long drive.

Good appointments this morning! Saw oncologist, doc-to-be, nurse, dietician, therapist, and Fredrica! Oncologist confirmed that I have my MRI on Friday and will receive my new round of chemo pills tomorrow. Dietician confirmed that I needed to make a few changes to my diet. (Yum…add back carbs!) Fredrica shared tips and supplements from her Herbalife program and lots of laughs (the best medicine), and the therapist confirmed that I'm just crazy enough to keep things interesting.

And now that my tummy is confirming that a fast-food burger may not have been my best choice, it's time to see my local doc about a little thyroid issue. (Seems I've flip-flopped; went from *hypo* to *hyper*.)

Anyone wanna come take a walk? It's 78 out right now albeit breezy!

Tess
January 12, 2017

In my relatively short "adventure" so far with cancer, I have learned so much. Truthfully, I feel like I've been a bit of a baby, letting the misery get to me sometimes. I feel especially shameful when I see what others have gone through in their journey.

On the other hand, the things I have learned about humanity will last a lifetime...and then hopefully through anyone else I (and you) may touch.

For example: During our recent trip to Nebraska, I tried to hide the embarrassment I felt over my physical weakness, but not one of our friends made me feel any less of a woman. They casually took turns helping me up and down, in and out—just reaching out a hand like I was royalty, not the dorky/damaged creature I felt like. They made me feel valuable. That I still belong on this earth.

Teresa, Fredrica, Tom, Kim, Terry, John, Kirk, Judy, Marie, and many others! Who have taken a moment of their day to see how mine is going.

Kayla, Tony, and Jesse, who live with me, day by day watching my changes and often being my heart, legs, hands, and eyes when mine don't want to work right. (Too many things going on at once with this old body! Ha!)

Mom, Nan, and Kayla, who gave up time in their own lives to come be my caretakers while I lived in Hope Lodge, bringing much-needed love and laughter.

The crew from Lubbock FOE who came to see me while "incarcerated" (LOL) and helped bring my mother down here to be with me—especially Jerry and Marie, who often went out of their way to check on me.

New friends (volunteers and patients) I met at the lodge and took time out of their days to show me kindness and friendship, Michelle, Becca, and Andrea.

The list goes on... It's important to me that you know I appreciate you and even more so, the difference you make in others' lives when you give a moment of your time. Sometimes, it's all the difference they need to face the challenges ahead and forge on through the battles.

We're human. We try not to focus on the little things like hair, weight, scars, etc...but when *you* look at someone and tell them, "I love you, and you're beautiful to me because I know your heart," you help remove or ease their fears and focus on the positive powers needed for healing.

When my daughter wraps her arms around me and says those things, I feel strong again. And when Tony looks into my eyes and wraps his arms around me and holds me tight, I feel whole again.

When *you* say you care (in whatever words), you help make all the difference in the world!

Never underestimate God's ability to use you (us) for beautiful things!

Isn't it amazing that we forget how wonderful, powerful, and *needed* we are...until we realize how we affect others?

Thank you for reminding me of all the goodness out there in the middle of an often chaotic and scary life! May every day bring you the joy, love, and laughter you have brought to me!

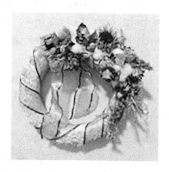

Tess
January 13, 2017

Good afternoon! I hope you all are having a great Friday the 13th!

You'll never believe it, but cold has finally arrived!

A wee bit of update:

1. Finally had my MRI this morning. I know I promised results...but I just got off the phone, and Doc is gone for the day. No results until next week.
2. Chemo pills have arrived. I will begin round two on Sunday. I decided it best to follow doctor's orders and see this through, but I also have an appointment locally on

Monday for an additional medication that I'm told will help with all the nasty side effects. (It may not stop me from losing the rest of my hair...but it may stop me from caring! LOL! It's okay. I've gotta laugh sometimes, and the best medicine is if you laugh with me!)

3. The wreath in the photo... I was going to give it a fancy name, but my creative thinker isn't working so well. Maybe you can come up with a name. It's in honor of the support shown to me through all this. First, I dried a flower from each arrangement I received while in the hospital. Second, our friend Jerry brought a box of "fresh cotton" (still in the pods from the field).

Mom had never been to Texas, nor had she seen cotton in the fields; so this was one of Jerry's normal friendly welcomes (he's always so thoughtful!). Mom took some home with her and left me some to be creative with.

So I bought a premade straw base and designed the cancer wreath. (Definitely not as pretty as the one Kim designed for us from the ribbons for when Tony and I exchanged vows.)

*****

I was finding some peace and joy in working with my hands again, and I began to feel almost normal! It was great to be home and sleeping in my own bed, helping out in my own kitchen, and even cleaning my own home. But I will say it again: I could not have done any of this without the American Cancer Society's Hope Lodge. What an amazing place it is! And if you have one in your neighborhood, call or go in and check them out, and see what needs they might have. If there isn't one in your area but you have cancer care and doctors, please consider contacting the American Cancer Society to see how you can help bring a Hope Lodge to your area.

*****

Tess
January 14, 2017

My first living-room slow dance in a loooooong time. Today hasn't been a good day physically, but that felt like an amazing blessing. (One of my favorite songs, "I'll Stand By You.")

*****

Don't skip these little moments if you can help it, and please don't discourage a patient from having them. They're a huge blessing in the realm of healing and, most importantly, in keeping the hope and faith alive.

I'm jumping ahead to 2018. Life on this journey has been beautiful at times and painful at others. Jesse Shane Brown passed away from the cancer and complications on Aug 30, 2018, not long after his 21st birthday. Losing a loved one to cancer is heartbreaking. It's painful knowing that a fellow warrior could no longer fight the battle.

Jesse had fought the enemy for more than ten years, and so many people loved and admired him. He fought bravely and maintained love and laughter for all those years. He had many dreams for his future; but toward the end, we all felt the loss of being unable to make some of them come true. Right until the end, he was one amazing warrior, who brought so much life and love to others.

*****

Tess
March 4, 2018

As I sit here at one of my doctor's offices, I reminisce about all life has brought and God's many blessings…and this man, I absolutely adore.

*****

He returned to work last week, and so provided a note to his coworkers, bosses, and HR.

*****

I have developed this note to let you know of all the things that have recently occurred in my life and to both offer and "vocalize" my family's appreciation for the wonderful things you have done for us.

In the summer of 2016, my then 19-year-old son, Jesse, was diagnosed with lung cancer (osteosarcoma from his previous disease at age 10 had metastasized to his lungs). The upper lobe of his right lung was removed at UMC, Lubbock, Texas.

A month later, my wife, Tess, was surprisingly diagnosed with brain cancer (anaplastic astrocytoma). She was operated on to remove the tumor and then prescribed 35 daily radiation treatments (seven weeks) in Lubbock, Texas, and followed by several months of pill-form chemotherapy at home in Hobbs.

During the summer of 2017, my now 20-year-old son was again diagnosed with lung cancer. He then wanted to be closer to his two older sisters in Idaho; so I personally moved him from Hobbs to Idaho Falls, Idaho, where after a twenty-hour surgery in Boise, the lower lobe of his right lung was removed.

In the spring of 2018, Jesse was again diagnosed with more sarcoma cancer. This time, the diagnosis was multiple thoracic tumors that were occluding his breathing and the return of blood flow to his heart. Radiation and immunotherapy were begun to improve his comfort. No more surgery was allowed, and soon, he reached his radiation limit as well.

Jesse kept his spirits up through the very end and was selected by the Greater Idaho Falls Chamber of Commerce as a "Distinguished Under 40 Honoree." He wanted to be an inspiration to those suffering from cancer. In the fall of 2018, two and one-half months after his 21st birthday, Jesse succumbed to cancer; and we lost him at the end of August.

Speaking for myself, a couple months later, at the beginning of November, I had a motorcycle accident breaking my back. I spent the next three weeks in intensive care at UMC, El Paso. At the end of November, I was released to return home and begin self-recovery. My injuries included a stable fracture of C-7; fracture and subsequent fusion of T-6, 7, 8, and 9 vertebrae; and fractured ribs 8–10.

After several months of physical recovery and healing, bi-weekly sessions of physical and speech therapy, at the end of February, I have returned to work on a part-time basis. Hopefully my physical and mental stamina will increase soon so I can return to full-time.

During all of these trials, many of you offered prayers, assistance, well wishes, visits, flowers, donations of gas money, and donations of vacation hours. I thank you very much. It was a tremendous offering, without which I'm not sure I would have mentally survived. WIPP, you are the best! And I count several of you close enough to say you are family. Thank you, thank you, thank you.

*****

Jesse
August 31, 2018

This is Jesse's sister Kelsie, posting on his behalf. If you are able to come support my baby brother's beautiful life celebration, we would very much appreciate it. There is a balloon release for him tomorrow at 7:00 p.m. in McCowin Park in Ammon and then a motorcycle escort after his services on Sunday to the Eagles Lodge. Hope to see you all!

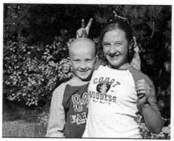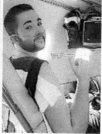